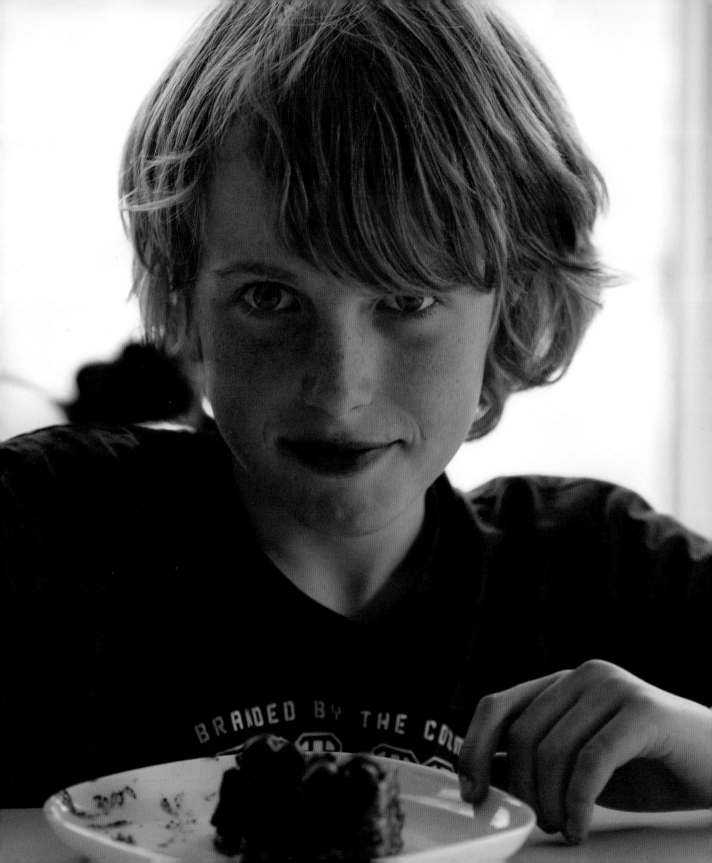

THE ART OF
RAW FOOD

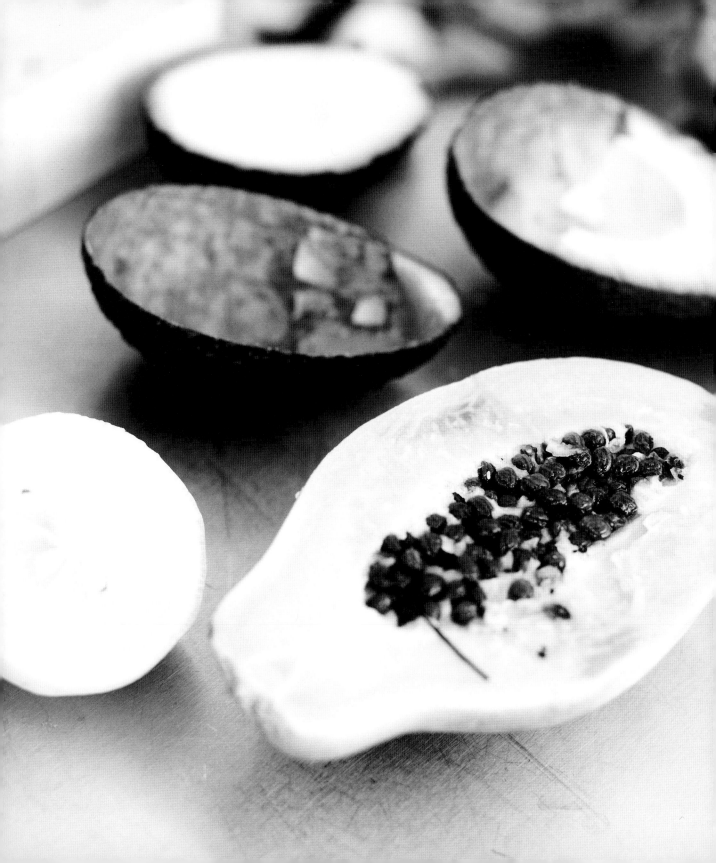

JENS CASUPEI   VIBEKE KAUPERT

THE ART OF
RAW FOOD

DELICIOUS, SIMPLE DISHES FOR HEALTHY LIVING

Foreword by David Wolfe

North Atlantic Books
Berkeley, California

Published by
North Atlantic Books
P.O. Box 12327
Berkeley, California 94712

Cover photo by Vibeke Kaupert
Cover design by Claudia Smelser
Book design by Vibeke Kaupert
Printed in the United States of America

First Danish edition published under the title *Raw Food* in 2009, Copenhagen, Denmark, by Thaning & Appel. ISBN: 9788741301723.

The Art of Raw Food: Delicious, Simple Dishes for Healthy Living is sponsored by the Society for the Study of Native Arts and Sciences, a nonprofit educational corporation whose goals are to develop an educational and cross-cultural perspective linking various scientific, social, and artistic fields; to nurture a holistic view of arts, sciences, humanities, and healing; and to publish and distribute literature on the relationship of mind, body, and nature.

North Atlantic Books' publications are available through most bookstores. For further information, visit our website at www.northatlanticbooks.com or call 800-733-3000.

MEDICAL DISCLAIMER: The following information is intended for general information purposes only. Individuals should always see their health care provider before administering any suggestions made in this book. Any application of the material set forth in the following pages is at the reader's discretion and is his or her sole responsibility.

Library of Congress Cataloging-in-Publication Data

Casupei, Jens, 1976–
 The art of raw food : delicious, simple dishes for healthy living / Jens Casupei, Vibeke Kaupert ; [foreword by] David Wolfe.
   p. cm.
Summary: Equally at home on the coffee table or in the kitchen, *The Art of Raw Food* features gorgeous four-color photography and delicious yet simple raw food recipes as well as a background on the benefits of a raw food diet. A terrific introduction to the world of raw foods for any newcomer, *The Art of Raw Food* offers 140 diverse and unique recipes sure to appeal to seasoned raw foodists as well."—Provided by publisher.

ISBN 978-1-58394-247-5 (hardback)
 1. Raw foods. 2. Vegetables. 3. Fruit. 4. Health. 5. Cookbooks. I. Kaupert, Vibeke, 1961- II. Title.
TX391.C37 2011
 641.5'636—dc22   2011002951

1 2 3 4 5 6 7 8 9   Sheridan   16 15 14 13 12 11

Foreword

I was first exposed to this beautiful Danish book while doing a detox cleanse and fast in Belgium. I was captivated by the pictures and the recipes. Normally, when such delicious cuisine is around (at a nearby raw food restaurant, for example), I will work hard and barely eat all day, knowing that in the evening my discipline will pay off with a well-earned, delightful meal. I had no such privilege or luxury during my cleanse in Belgium. All I could do was peruse the wonderful recipes found within these pages and imagine tasting and testing them, so instead I delved into the book's more introductory and informational aspects.

As Jens and Vibeke point out, raw food lessens our deleterious impact on our immune systems, our communities, our nations, and our planet. Raw food is environmentally friendly, sustainable, simple, fun, innovative, trendy, and is the future! What a combination! As the problems and challenges in our world continue to mount, the solutions continue to present themselves. Raw food is part of a holistic solution to our world's ills.

The Art of Raw Food delivers a practical guide to understanding the idea of a raw food diet as well as to preparing uncooked, plant-based cuisine. Jens and Vibeke artistically deliver a menu that is rich in cancer-fighting and heart-healthy fruits, vegetables, nuts, seeds, seaweeds, sprouts, herbs, and even some superfoods! Recipe instructions are clear enough even for children to learn how to make the imaginative dishes found within these pages. *The Art of Raw Food* is definitely for the entire family to enjoy.

I'm always excited to support an increasingly popular book in the raw food genre, especially a book with such extraordinary recipes and beautiful photos! *The Art of Raw Food* is the first raw food book since Kristine Nolfi's *Raw Food Treatment of Cancer* (nearly seventy years ago) that has made its way over from Denmark to North America.

Enjoy *The Art of Raw Food!*

And…Have the Best Day Ever!!!

David Wolfe (www.davidwolfe.com), founder of the nonprofit Fruit Tree Planting Foundation (ftpf.org), author of *The Sunfood Diet Success System, Eating for Beauty, Superfoods, Naked Chocolate,* and *Amazing Grace.*

November 2010

Preface

I wrote this book out of my love for food and a desire to live life to the fullest while enjoying it as much as possible. The food you will read about in *The Art of Raw Food* will give you energy and time to enjoy life. It is seductive food that tastes delicious, food that brings the best tastes out of ingredients.

Sometimes food should be quick and easy to prepare. At other times I personally enjoy the challenge of preparing great food. Regardless, for me preparing food must be fun and the final result should enchant my guests. Food should enliven the senses and stimulate our passion for life. Food should be amazing and delicious, simple and raw. All the recipes in this book are easy to make, down-to-earth, and uncomplicated. It is all about getting down to basics—down to the clean and pure enjoyment of food.

When writing this book, I reverted to a very basic question, a question that has lingered in the back of my mind at various stages of my life: Does it enrich me?

In the case of this book: Does it enrich my life to eat raw food? Does it taste divine? Do I crave it? Will my body be full of energy when I eat?

For me the answer to all these questions is YES!

I love raw food. I hope this book will show you why and make you want to try raw food.

Enjoy!

Jens Casupei

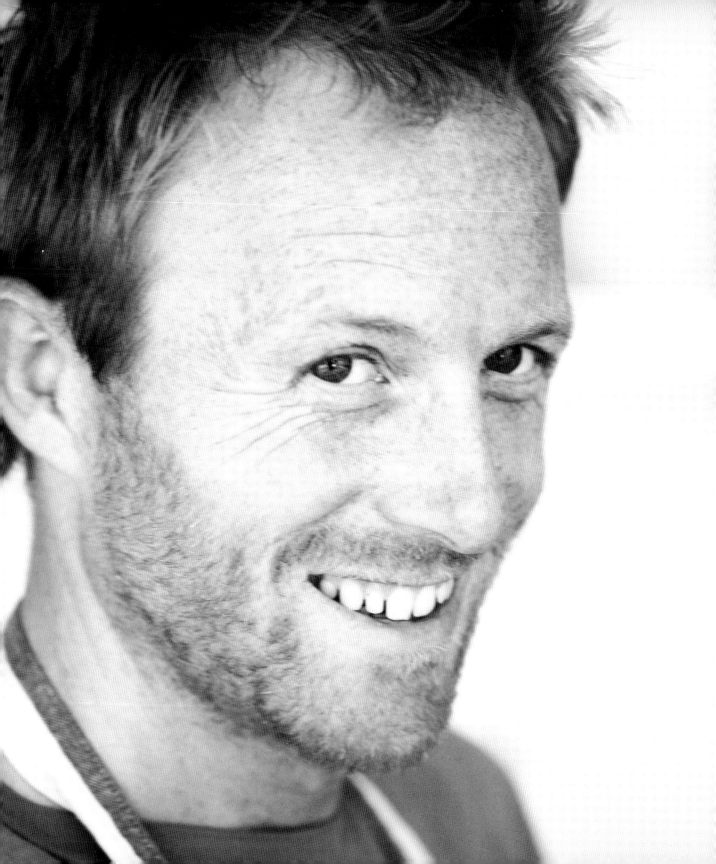

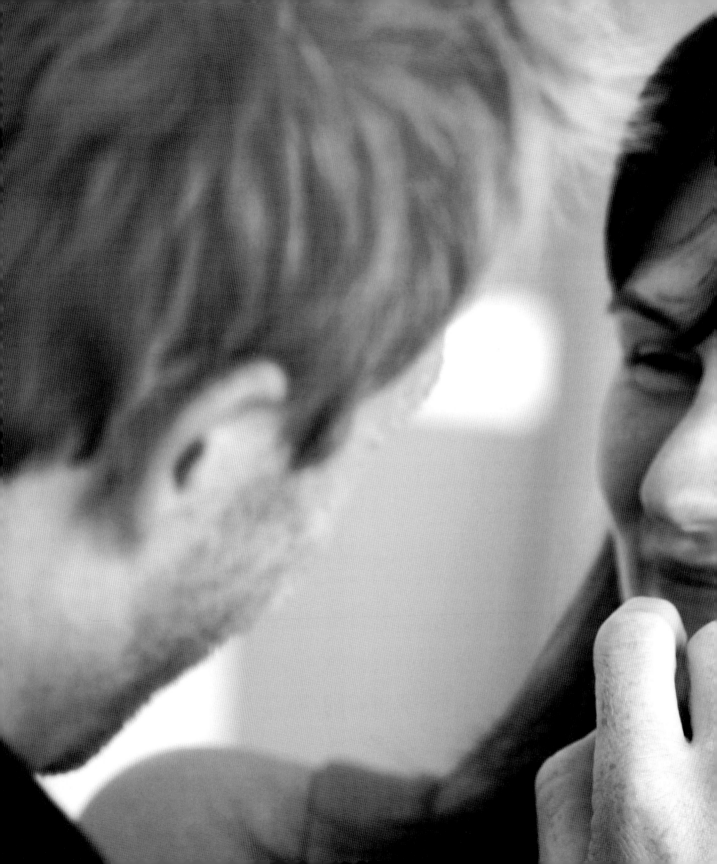

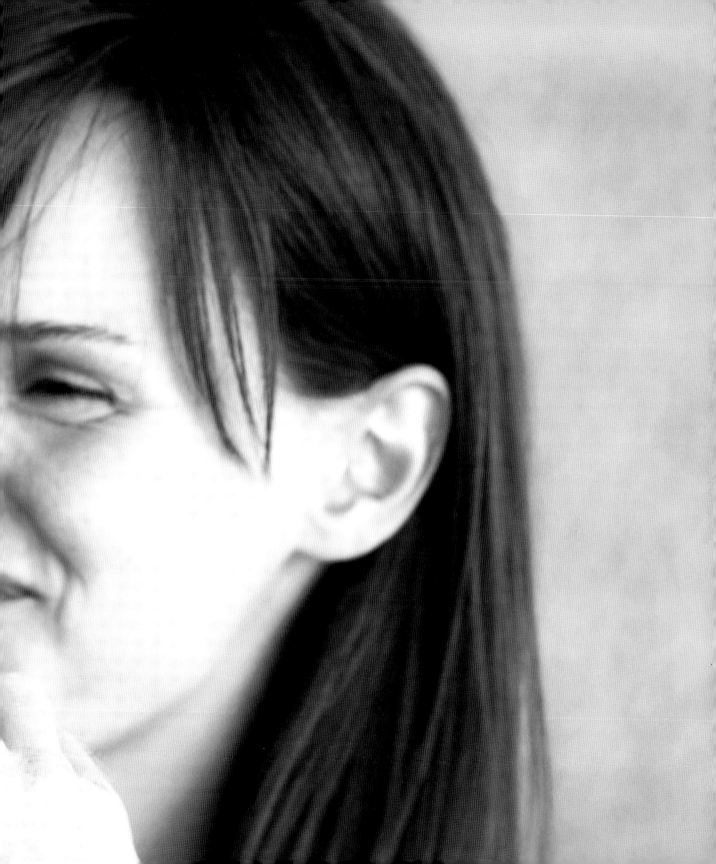

Contents

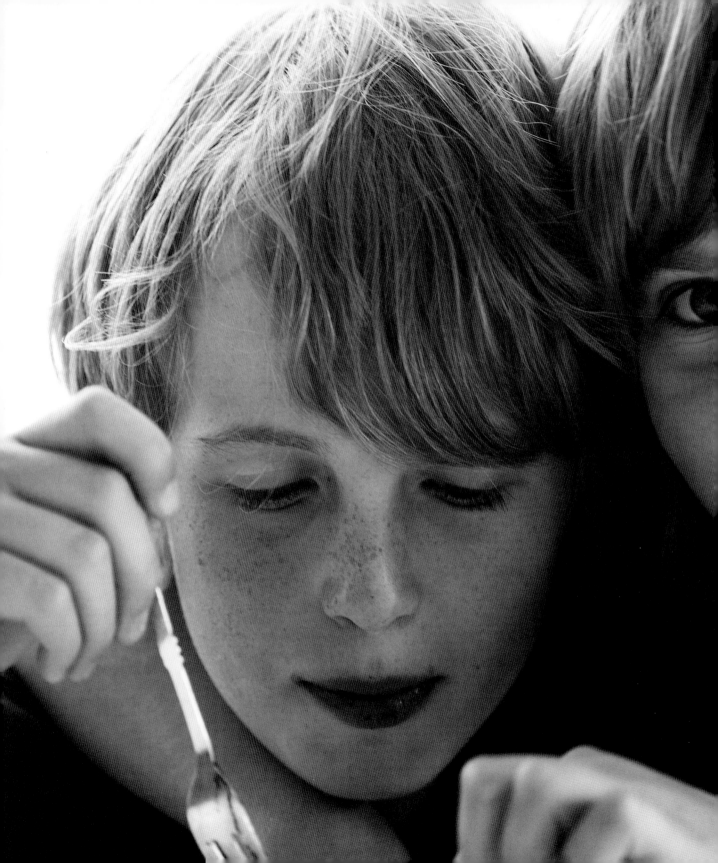

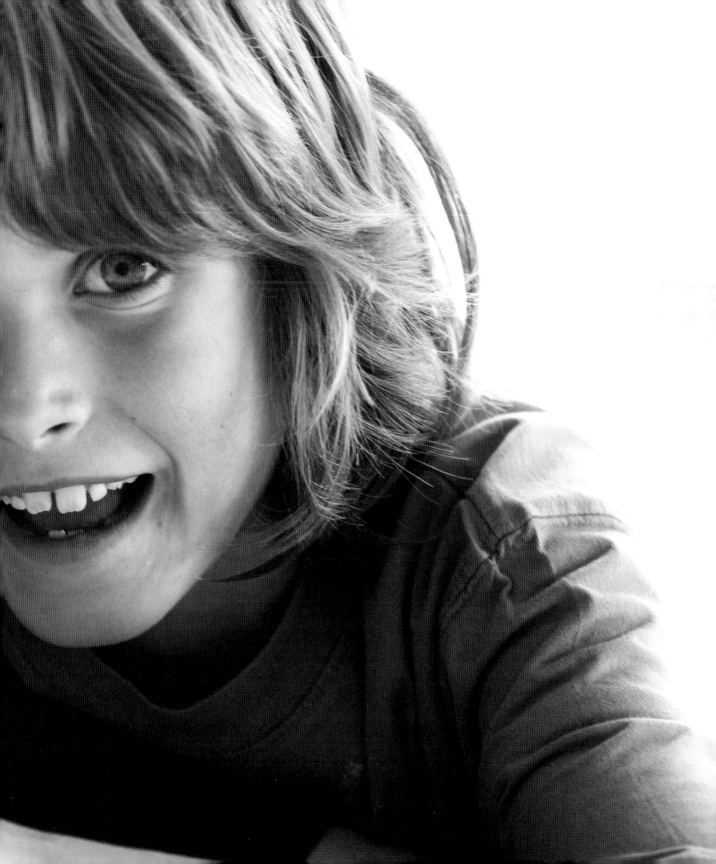

Raw Food Overview

Why Read This Book?

There are two reasons why I wrote this book. Firstly, my job involves helping people to be happy, get healthy, and live the life they have always dreamed of. I have discovered the unequivocal benefits of raw food in helping my clients achieve these goals. Regardless of who you are, what you do, or what your current situation is, you can achieve substantial improvements through a raw food diet: physically, mentally, and emotionally.

Secondly, in writing this book, I strive to share my passion with you. I love food and I love life. Food must be heavenly delicious and life must be lived to the full. For me, raw food is the best way to achieve both. I have added beautiful pictures of every dish in the book so you can see how delicate, exquisite, and sexy raw food can be.

My objective is to inspire you and arouse your curiosity; to awaken your desire to try raw food, which will give you the ultimate rush of vitality in your body. I want you to experience the fantastic benefits of eating raw food:

- You will be more radiant and healthy.
- You will think more clearly.
- You will have more energy to do the things you truly enjoy.
- You will be happier.
- You will rid yourself of physical ailments.

You don't have to be a gourmet cook or a pastry chef to be able to make the dishes in this book. Even people who have never tried to cook before have told me how much fun they have had and how easy it was for them to follow the recipes.

I am keenly aware that there is not just one universal truth and I do not in any way claim to have all the answers. This book includes my personal views and ideas and is intended as a source of inspiration.

Raw food is raw and unprocessed food. It is plant-based and filled with life-force nutrients and energy. With raw food you will experience an abundance of color, texture, and taste that is unsurpassed in other cuisines. Raw food brings out the ultimate character of each ingredient. Raw food can be described as creamy, crisp, juicy, lush, strong, sweet, light, crunchy, and extremely tasty. It is food that focuses on enchanting your eyes, palate, and nose. You will not need to count calories with raw food, but bite-by-bite, you will fill your body with health and vitality. Raw food contains enzymes, vitamins, and other nutrients that are perfectly balanced and in sync with your body since they have not been destroyed by heating or other forms of processing. Raw food is food in its purest and most natural form.

Enzymes can rightfully be called the fountain of youth. They are necessary for breaking down and absorbing the food you eat. Enzymes are essential for the body's vitality. The fewer enzymes in food, the less vitality it contains. The same applies to your body. Heating food to over 118 degrees Fahrenheit destroys the enzymes present in the raw ingredients. Food that contains few or no enzymes depletes your body of its own natural resources, accelerates the aging process, and causes illness. Raw food, on the other hand, enhances your natural beauty, health, and intelligence while slowing down the aging process.

> "So what was the biggest change for me? Normally I feel myself aging day by day. Now I feel younger each day that passes." (Matthew Kenney, raw food gourmet cook).

Raw food is for everyone, regardless of taste preferences. It includes lasagna, chili stews, strawberry smoothies, creamy soups, easy salads, carrot cakes, blueberry pies, and lots and lots of chocolate. You can go raw at all meals—breakfast, lunch, and dinner—as well as for snack times during the day. These recipes are easy and can make anyone prepare food like a gourmet cook. And perhaps the best fun of going raw is that you will never have to worry again about burning your food!

Raw food is not new. Before we discovered fire and started cooking our food, we ate everything raw. Humans are in fact the only species on Earth to heat food. All other creatures eat raw food.

Raw Food: A History

Raw food is both new and ancient. It has also been called "light food" and "living food." Several trends exist within the raw food movement, with a common denominator: the belief that our diet should consist of as many raw vegetables and fruits as possible, and that they should be consumed in an unadulterated state.

In the millennia since humans first discovered fire and began cooking, the oldest evidence of a raw food diet dates back to ancient Greece. Pythagoras established a philosophical, mathematical, and spiritual school in which the inner circle, known as *mathematikoi,* together with Pythagoras, were vegans and ate raw food. Another renowned thinker from ancient Greece is Hippocrates, father of modern medicine and creator of the original oath that all doctors take today, the Hippocratic oath. One of his famous quotes is "Let food be your medicine." There is strong indication that he too lived mainly on raw food, as he, like Pythagoras and *mathematikoi,* believed that doing so was optimal for health and intellectual ability.

The raw food movement as we know it today took off in the United States at the beginning of the twenty-first century. Juliano and other raw food gourmet chefs captured the attention of the media and Hollywood stars with colorful, delicious dishes with an intense taste experience. Celebrities quickly adopted the new cuisine, which, besides being innovative, trendy, and delicate, helped them feel younger and fitter.

Eating raw soon became a hot trend. It was exquisite gourmet food, and one could eat as much as desired without worrying about calories. The diet removed excess weight and reduced wrinkles. Glowing skin and sparkling eyes were back. The taste was sinful and the result healthy. Modern and stylish restaurants popped up in big cities, while several books on raw food were published.

At the same time, the growing and increasingly influential alternative health movement focused passionately on the influence of nutrition on everything from health to state of mind, to beauty and physical ability. Again and again, raw food was lauded as optimal for our health and spiritual development, enhancing intelligence, curing illnesses, and for improving quality of life.

It was not only in the alternative health sector that raw food gained popularity. Doctors, psychologists, and researchers all over the world had already utilized raw food to cure themselves and their patients of cancer,

Alzheimer's, and similar diseases. The term "mood foods" was also used due to the strong influence raw food has on our mood and mental state. It was all about eating our way to health and happiness, freed from depression and illness.

Just after World War II, the Danish physician Kristine Nolfi cured herself of breast cancer by eating only raw vegetables and fruit. Similar stories can be found from all over the world. In 1993, Dr. Lorraine Day, head of the orthopedic surgery department at San Francisco General Hospital, was diagnosed with breast cancer. The verdict was terminal breast cancer. However, by switching over to raw food, she was totally cured without the need for chemotherapy or radiation treatments.

Hollywood Goes Raw

Actresses such as Uma Thurman, Lisa Bonet, Angela Bassett, Daryl Hannah, and Susan Sarandon have talked about incorporating raw food principles in their kitchens.

The men of Hollywood have also joined in: among others, Robin Williams, Woody Harrelson, Jared Leto, Edward Norton, and Pierce Brosnan. Radio personality Howard Stern has also expressed his passion for raw food.

The fashion and glamour world has taken to the principles of eating raw food as well. Former supermodel Carol Alt wrote the book *Eating in the Raw: A Beginner's Guide to Getting Slimmer, Feeling Healthier, and Looking Younger the Raw-Food Way.* In the book, she reflects on her youth and how she starved herself in order to stay thin and as a consequence developed serious health issues. Today, she eats only raw food and has never looked better.

Fashion icon Donna Karan has also switched to raw food. After losing almost 22 pounds by eating raw food, she decided to spread the word to others. She spoke candidly about her experience of eating raw food on *The Martha Stewart Show.*

From the music business, Sting, David Bowie, and Anthony Kiedis from the Red Hot Chili Peppers have started eating raw food as well.

The father of life coaching, Anthony Robbins, who has coached tennis stars such as Serena Williams and Andre Agassi and has served as a personal adviser to President Bill Clinton, is also a dedicated raw food advocate.

Raw Food and Athletes

Can you eat raw food and still build muscle and perform sports at a high level?

After twenty years of inactivity, at the age of thirty-seven, Tim VanOrden started his career as a raw food athlete. Within a very short period on his raw food diet, Tim realized that he had discovered something big. In record time, he trained himself to become one of the best mountain runners in California, winning several competitions.

Now he also participates in competitions that involve running as fast as possible to the top of some of the world's tallest skyscrapers. In 2008, he won the U.S. Bank Tower Stair Climb, where he set a new record by running up each and every step to the seventy-fifth floor. But regardless of whether he runs up mountains, up stairs, or plows his way through knee-high powder wearing a pair of snowshoes, he manages to outrun competitors twenty years younger than he. In all three disciplines, he is considered to be among the elite, even though he is over forty years of age.

> "A change to a raw vegan diet was the best decision I ever made as an athlete. My stamina has improved dramatically and I am able to recuperate from hard training and competitions in half the normal time. I have had to stop weight training at the gym because I am now building muscle at a much faster rate than before, which makes me a slower runner. My asthma is gone, and I no longer suffer from joint pain." (Tim VanOrden, *Running Raw*).

Brendan Brazier is yet another sports star who has endorsed raw food. He started eating raw food in order to cope with fatigue and chronic muscle pains. He is a two-time Canadian champion of the 50-kilometer Ultramarathon, in 2003 and 2006. Moreover, he is a professional Ironman triathlete, who time and again triumphs over his competitors. He is an established writer and speaker and sports nutrition expert and has twice been invited to speak to the U.S. House of Representatives about the socioeconomic advantages of improving personal health through healthy eating habits.

One of the United States' best cyclists, Bob Mionske, who won over forty-five bicycle races in his career, attributes much of his success to eating raw food. He describes it as a natural development for a healthy lifestyle. Bob represented the United States in the 1988 Summer Olympics in Seoul, South Korea, where he made the winning break in the men's Individual Road Race, finishing in fourth place, and two years later he won the U.S. National Championship in the men's road race.

Savate (a French version of kickboxing) expert James Southwood has called the raw food lifestyle "an easy, pure, and wholesome way of living. Training and competing in this physical state is the only way I would ever choose." Southwood is the British Champion (2006, 2008), European Vice Champion, and World Bronze medalist in Savate.

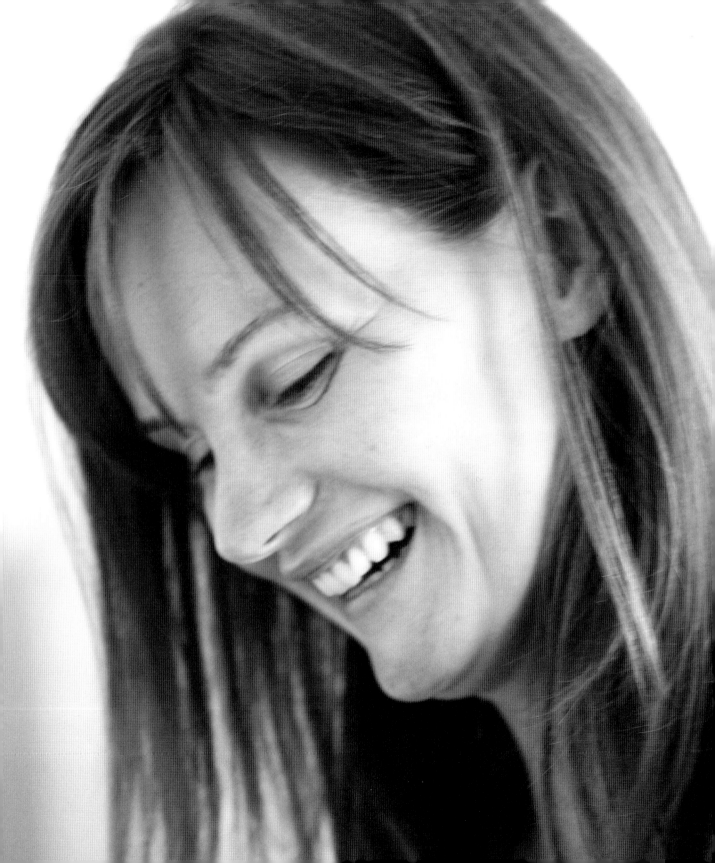

Raw Food = Raw Muscle Power

Peter Ragnar is a good example of how raw food and raw power go hand in hand. In August 2004, he did a thousand push-ups in twenty-three minutes. With the tips of the fingers of one hand, he has managed to lift seven weight discs weighing a total of 165 pounds. This feat earned him an unofficial world record. Considering that Peter had long since passed retirement age when he demonstarted these abilities, his prowess is truly impressive.

Dr. Gabriel Cousens, MD, MD(H), DD, founder and director of The Tree of Life Rejuvenation Center, is a leading author and world-renowned spiritual teacher and expert in raw, living-food nutrition and healing. On his sixtieth birthday, he performed six hundred consecutive push-ups for his guests. I am not sure if he did it to inspire his guests to experience how much energy they would derive from eating the raw chocolate cake, but how many people do you know who can do six hundred push-ups?

Performing such impressive feats on a diet of raw food is not limited only to humans. With one arm, chimpanzees can rip your car door off, and a gorilla, which is ten times as strong as a human, can lift more than two tons. Both primates, who are our closest relatives, live entirely on raw food—and thrive on it.

These are just a few examples of the exceptional physical performance that is possible on a raw food diet. Discover the possibilities for yourself!

Raw Food: The Technical Details

Definition

A raw food diet is the closest we can get to the original human diet, a source of invigorating, life-giving nutrients. Raw food, prepared without heating to above 118 degrees Fahrenheit, is made of organic ingredients in their most natural form, and includes all the nutrients you need in order to help you live a healthy life full of energy. Raw food is the most nutritious and vital food you can eat. It is food that enhances beauty, health, and intelligence.

Raw food in its most seductive form offers gourmet dishes that will make your mouth water and arouse your senses. In its simplest form, it could be a slice of melon, a handful of sun-ripened blackberries, or a freshly dug up carrot. Regardless of how you prefer it, it is irresistible.

> "You need not be a vegetable guru or a health freak to be able to appreciate the benefits of raw food. As most of us know, all life-forms die at 109 degrees Fahrenheit: cats, dogs, humans—and food. Raw food is much bet-

ter for the body and for the digestive system. The higher the level of enzymes found in food, the more benefit we can get out of it. And it can be delicious and satisfying gourmet food at the same time." (Pierre Spiridon, Swedish master chef, and food pioneer).

The Importance of Enzymes

Enzymes are charged protein molecules that control the biomechanical processes in your body's metabolism. All vital processes in your body are dependent on enzymes. Enzymes are responsible for every chemical reaction in each and every cell of your body. Minerals, vitamins, and hormones cannot function without enzymes. You would not be able to lift your arm above your head or even think without the presence of enzymes.

Food that is heated to a temperature of less than 118 degrees Fahrenheit contains enzymes that assist your digestive system in breaking down food into its components, thus enabling your body to absorb essential nutrients. These enzymes are activated as soon as you take your first bite of food, and they go on to break down the food's cellular membrane. When you eat raw food, you do not deplete your body's own stock of enzymes—these can be used instead to keep you young and healthy. You will get a lot of energy from the food passing through your digestive system without leaving any undesirable residues that can lodge in your bowels for several years.

Biological Enzymes Are the Source of All Life in Your Body

Enzymes are essential both for your digestion and for your body's own rejuvenation process. They are nature's detoxifying agents, cleansing your body of both interior and exterior pollutants. Enzymes aid the repair of your DNA and RNA while maintaining and strengthening your immune system. They transform and store energy in your body; they break down fibers. Enzymes are anti-inflammatory agents that have a pain-relieving capacity and counteract water retention in the body. Enzymes are also beneficial in minimizing the consequences of injuries and reducing the recuperation period from sports and other types of activities.

Enzymes are essential for maintaining a healthy and youthful body. Dr. Edward Howell, one of America's pioneers in the study of enzymes' role in food and our bodies, has stated that the amount of enzymes in our bodies equals what we call our life force or vitality. He considers the body's enzyme levels a good indicator of our state of health. The amount of enzymes measured in the saliva of an average twenty-five-year-old is almost thirty times higher than that of an average eighty-one-year-old. After a long period of chronic illness, a person's enzyme levels are usually very low. Put simply, your body's enzyme reserves can be compared to a battery. You can recharge it or you can drain it, all depending on what you eat. When your enzyme levels are high, you have energy and all your body functions perform optimally. If the level falls, your body functions slowly start to shut down and you get older—regardless of your chronological age.

"As the amount of enzymes in our bodies diminishes with age, so does our ability to perform various functions that are instrumental in keeping our body healthy. The aging process occurs when the enzyme concentration in the body diminishes." (Gabriel Cousens).

So if you want to stay youthful and maintain your natural beauty and energy, it is of paramount importance that you eat food with a high concentration of enzymes while avoiding food that steals your energy and drains your body of vital enzymes.

You can improve the natural amount of enzymes in your body by eating enzyme-rich foods because the excess enzymes will be absorbed into your body's enzyme deposits, from where they can be circulated through the body and perform vital processes. Raw and unprocessed food naturally contains a high level of enzymes, which in turn lead to increased physical stamina and energy, to a positive outlook on life, and to good health. You can thus achieve a youthful body and mind regardless of your age. You can live with the energy of a twenty-year-old even though you have reached your sixties.

What Raw Food Is Not

Raw food is not pasteurized, gene-modified, processed, cooked, fried, baked, sprayed, microwaved, or chemically treated food. It is without artificial additives or inscrutable E numbers (number codes for additives, commonly found on food labels within the European Union).

When Foods Become Harmful: The Effect of Heating Food

Heated and processed food has a very low or even nonexistent level of vital enzymes. Heating food reduces its nutritional value and at the same time damages certain substances in food, thus making them harmful to your body.

During the process of heating, for example while frying, boiling, or baking, the enzymes in food are destroyed. The food you subsequently put in your mouth includes few or no enzymes, so your body is obliged to use its own stores to process the intake of food. Your enzyme reserves are thus depleted in the process of consuming heated food.

This depletion can have far-reaching consequences and may be the cause of various illnesses, depression, apathy, reduced mental performance, and reduced energy—conditions that are often associated with aging, but could also perhaps just be your body's way of signaling that you are enzyme deficient.

Heating does not merely destroy essential enzymes; it also destroys active forms of vitamins and minerals. Almost 85 percent of all nutritional value in food is thus destroyed through heating.

According to the Max Planck Institute, 50 percent of proteins found in food coagulate when heated. This makes it more difficult for the body to break down proteins into vital amino acids, limiting the body's absorption of proteins consumed.

Not only does heating reduce food's nutritional value, in some instances it can also cause vital amino acids and fatty acids to be transformed into substances that are extremely harmful to your body. Cooking creates a high level of free radicals in food. Excessive amounts of free radicals in the body can lead to cell injury and death, resulting in diseases such as cancer, stroke, myocardial infarction, diabetes, and other major disorders. It can also cause premature aging. Furthermore, certain types of naturally occurring substances, which in their raw food form are responsible for combating undesired organisms and fungicides, become transformed by heating into toxic chemical components.

In April 2002, scientists at Stockholm University discovered that baking, frying, roasting, and deep-frying foodstuffs containing high levels of carbohydrates led to an undesired by-product know as acrylamide. This chemical compound damages both the central and the peripheral nervous system and can potentially be carcinogenic.

The study showed that a bag of potato chips could contain five hundred times more acrylamide than the levels recommended for drinking water by the World Health Organization (WHO). Foods that typically include large amounts of this substance are baked potatoes, chips, bread, cookies, and other high-carbohydrate baked goods.

Dr. William Newsome of Canada's Department of Health and Welfare Food Research Division, Bureau of Chemical Safety, made another discovery. In samples of heated food, he found over fifty times more ETU—a mutation and carcinogenic agent—than that found in nonheated food. In some instances, cooked tomatoes contained over ninety times more ETU.

Heating food weakens the nutritional properties of what you eat and creates toxic substances and harmful compounds that can cause your body to deteriorate and ultimately lead to serious illnesses and other adverse health conditions.

Perhaps you may have been told how important it is to heat your food in order to kill germs and bacteria, and by doing so avoid getting sick from the food you eat. I, however, would argue for the exact opposite; yes, heating does in fact kill bacteria, but heating also destroys the enzymes and vitamins contained in your food. Devoid of enzymes and vitamins, your immune system cannot perform its primary function of protecting you against harmful viruses and bacteria. Moreover, there are strong indicators that if your body is not exposed to bacteria, you run a much higher risk of developing allergies.

The Effects of Processed Food

The "chromium effect" is a good example of how processed food can affect our bodies. Chromium is a mineral that is instrumental in balancing the body's blood sugar levels. It plays an important role in the production of insulin and the formation of good cholesterol in the body, and also has an effect on the synthesis between protein and RNA.

Raw and unprocessed brown sugar and corn both contain the required amounts of the mineral chromium to ensure the absorption of carbohydrates in the body. Conversely, processed white sugar and flour contain far lower levels of this mineral. When you eat white sugar and flour, you force your body to utilize its own storage of chromium in order to absorb carbohydrates. In the long term, this can lead to chromium deficiency in the body and can cause various illnesses.

Your Body at War with Food

Your body's natural reaction to viruses, infections, stress, and other toxic invaders that threaten your health is to immediately increase the production of white blood cells. These cells rush to the afflicted area, where they combat and neutralize the invading foe.

The same process occurs when you eat food that is heated, refined, preserved, homogenized, pasteurized, or in any other way processed. Your body considers this type of food to be harmful and combats it in the same way it fights against the flu virus or any other harmful agent. The process entails channeling white blood cells from your blood and immune system to your stomach in order to combat the intrusive element posing a threat to your health.

For many years it was thought that this was a natural process, termed "digestive leukocytosis." Subsequent scientific studies have not been able to confirm this phenomenon. In fact, it is unnecessary and stressful condition that puts your system on high alert, wearing your body out and causing it to deteriorate.

When you eat raw and unprocessed food this process does not occur. Your body instinctively recognizes raw food as nutrition and thus is not subjected to undue stress. The number of white blood cells does not increase. At the same time, your immune system remains strong and ready to eliminate diseases and fight other threats to your health.

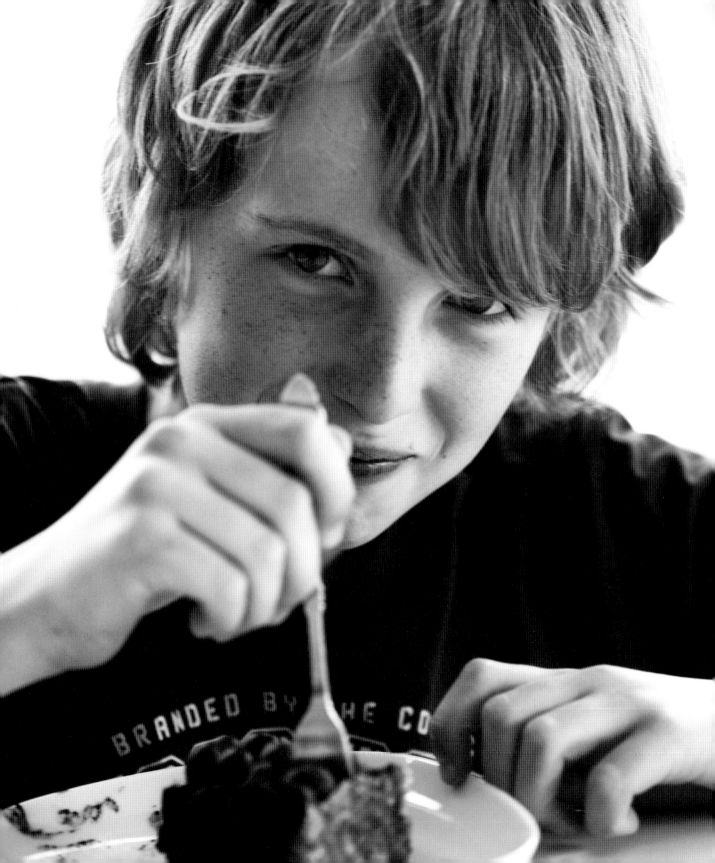

Avoiding Lifestyle Diseases

Would you like to minimize your risk of contracting today's major killers and lifestyle diseases?

From 1932 to 1942, Dr. Francis Pottenger, MD, studied the effects of heated and processed food versus raw and unprocessed foods. The results of his studies were astounding. In his classic experiments studying the effect of diet on cats, more than nine hundred cats were observed. Dr. Pottenger found that only diets containing raw and unprocessed foods produced optimal health. After ten years and three generations, the cats that were fed raw and unprocessed foods were healthy, while the cats that had been fed heated and processed foods were unable to reproduce, were deformed, and had several life-threatening diseases.

His findings were disturbing. Initially it may seem difficult to compare humans to cats; but it is nevertheless interesting to note that the diseases the cats contracted are seen more and more in humans. In fact, all the diseases observed in the cats were normally only associated with humans. The only thing that separated the sick cats from the healthy ones was the diet they were fed. What would that mean if the same were applied to you and me?

We are the only species on Earth that eats heated and processed food. This should be considered in light of the fact that we are the only species that suffers from cardiovascular diseases, osteoporosis, obesity, nutrition-related depressions, Alzheimer's, and many other ailments. We encounter these ailments only in domesticated animals and wild animals in captivity—in other words, animals that are fed heated and processed foods. All diseases that constitute the major killers of humans are those whose origins are obscure and that are not contracted by animals living in the wild.

Food is probably not the only cause of these extremely unpleasant diseases. Pollution, stress, poor sleep quality, and other factors have an impact. But what if you could substantially reduce your own risk for these serious diseases and illnesses by simply changing your eating habits?

Slim and Healthy with Raw Food

Discover the easiest, smartest, and most natural way to get slim. You won't need to count calories or even control portions. You can eat all you like until you are full and satisfied.

To be slim, healthy, and beautiful is natural, what nature intended you to be. That is the only thing you need to know in order to get the body you have always dreamed of.

Your body knows exactly what is required and how much. It is merely waiting for you to take the first step toward the change that will render you the radiant, beautiful, and fit person you have always wanted to be. You don't need to read any books, attend any seminars, starve yourself, or follow difficult diet plans.

If you just give your body the optimal conditions, it will automatically return to its natural weight and health. If you give your body what it needs in order to minimize or eradicate all that is harmful to you, your body will give you the life you have always wanted.

Models and fashion icons have already embraced this simple recipe for getting their natural beauty back. As mentioned before, Donna Karan lost 22 pounds just by switching to raw food. Former supermodel Carol Alt, voted one of the most beautiful women in the world, is now, at age fifty, even slimmer and in better shape than she was in her twenties. She describes her health as optimal and says she feels full of energy and enjoys having gotten rid of many ailments and physiological disorders—all thanks to eating a raw food diet.

Stories abound from people who have shed pounds and experienced the fabulous results of eating raw food. In its Fit Nation campaign, CNN told the story of Angela Stokes, who lost 165 pounds in just two years. She had never before had the desire to change her eating habits, as food was her only source of enjoyment. But things changed for her with raw food. She managed to satisfy her need for indulgence while enjoying the feeling of being physically satiated. She had no regrets after making the transition, and after the first month on a raw food diet, she met her first boyfriend in over five years. In the ensuing period she experienced dramatic changes emotionally, physically, and socially. She regained her appetite for life and says she has never felt happier: "Raw food changed my life completely."

Let Your Body Do the Work for You

Whether you weigh just a few pounds too much or carry a great deal of weight, it is not a problem. On the contrary, the extra fat has good reason to be there. It is one of nature's wonderful inventions, created to ensure that you stay alive.

Obesity actually has a double function: it has a protective element to it as well as a warning mechanism. Obesity tells you that you are out of balance, while at the same time protecting you from the consequences of that imbalance. You will begin to understand your body differently once you start viewing excess fat in this way, and will find it easier to achieve your ideal body weight again. You can begin to work with your body and follow some simple rules instead of fighting against them. Your body is always ready and alert, willing to help you as soon as you give it the go-ahead signal.

Your body is unique and wondrous. It processes millions of pieces of information, functions each and every second, and is highly skilled at doing so. Your consciousness is only a small part of your body's enormous knowledge and skill. The qualities and abilities you can handle with your conscious mind are impressive, but they can't compare to what your body can perform. From splitting your DNA to sustaining your physical and mental functions, your body has total control. It has since you were conceived.

Become your body's best friend and it will help you stay young, healthy, and radiant. The best you can do is let your body take over for you.

Eat All You Want and Lose Weight

Imagine being able to eat all you want, as much as you want, and whenever you so desire, without putting on one ounce. Imagine eating a big piece of chocolate cake and knowing that your body will benefit from it and that you will lead your body to its ideal weight. That is one of the advantages of raw food.

You will start needing less and less food once your body gets accustomed to eating raw. You will naturally start craving healthier alternatives and you will instinctively know what you need and desire. You will most likely become happier, have more energy and less need to resort to comfort eating or overeating.

If you have a bit too much body fat when you start eating raw food, you should expect to lose about 4 to 5 pounds during the first week. Over a longer period, it is quite normal to lose about 2 pounds per week.

If you are already slim, you may not experience much weight change, but you will most surely find it easier to build muscle and your body will become better proportioned.

Your Body Functions as a Whole

An imbalance in your weight cannot be seen as an isolated issue. All the functions of your body are connected, and a change in one system can influence the rest of the body. Your weight is thus the result of what goes on in your glands, your lungs, your digestive system, your liver, your heart, and your blood. Moreover, your sleep habits, thoughts, and level of stress and activity are also influential. You can experience bringing all these functions into alignment and balance once you switch to eating raw and unprocessed food. The benefits are thus for your entire body and not just for achieving weight loss.

Weight and Enzymes

When taking a closer look at the biological mechanisms in your body and the reasons for being overweight, two enzyme groups stand out: proteases and lipases.

Proteases are a group of enzymes that are crucial for sustaining optimal health. Proteases aid in the breaking down of proteins and amino acids while removing various toxic substances. Your body's ability to remove these toxic substances is essential for the fat-burning process. If you are unable to remove these toxins, your body stores them in fat in order to ensure that they do not cause harm. It is your body's way of protecting you from the adverse effects of the toxins. This means that you will put on weight and it becomes almost impossible to shed the excess pounds. Regardless of how much you exercise or reduce fat intake in your diet, your body will simply refuse to get rid of the fat until it has a sufficient level of proteases.

Eating lots of fruit and vegetables supplies your body with large amounts of proteases. This results in your body again being able to expel toxins since they now can be neutralized. The process will ultimately lead to reducing the amount of body fat required to encapsulate harmful substances. Your body will automatically burn fat when it has sufficient stores of proteases.

Lipases, which are found in great quantities in raw food, are a group of fatty acid degradation enzymes. If you eat heated food, you are probably not getting sufficient amounts of lipases through your diet, since enzymes are destroyed by heating or processing. Eating heated food can thus result in difficulties with burning the fat you eat, not to mention getting rid of all the excess fat you carry. Lipases aid in the processes of digesting, distributing, and fat burning. Lipases break down and dissolve fat in your body. Without lipases, fat accumulates in your body. It is this fat that you may see on your hips, your thighs, your behind, and your stomach. So in short, enzymes such as lipases and proteases play a crucial role in your attempt to lose weight or stay fit.

Break the Vicious Circle: Malnourishment, Overeating, and Fat Accumulation

If you eat food with low or no nutritional value, it is quite likely that you will end up in a vicious cycle of malnourishment, overeating, and fat accumulation. Your stomach is not much bigger than a clenched fist. If you feel that you need to eat bigger quantities than that in order to feel satiated, you are at risk of ending up in that vicious cycle.

The prime reason for eating is to get energy and nutrition for the thousands of processes that take place in your body every second. You eat to live. When your body needs replenishment, it sends a hunger signal to your brain. When you consume the nourishment you need, the hunger signal stops.

However, when you eat food that does not contain sufficient nutrients, your body continues to signal to you that you are hungry and you end up overeating. When your stomach is more than filled, your body starts to send a new type of signal. This says that the body now has to start storing fat in order to be ready for meager times that may come. The obvious result of this process is that you start to put on weight. Your body keeps sending out signals that it is hungry even though you are gaining weight. This is the vicious cycle that you need to break.

If you continue to eat food with low nutritional value, you just continue the above scenario. You can reduce your portions and avoid eating cakes and desserts for long periods without losing any weight. It could even be that by just tasting something that is a little bit sweet you start accumulating more fat. It all seems like a hopeless situation but the solution is just as effective as it is simple.

When you eat food filled with enzymes, vitamins, minerals, and other nutritional elements, your body finally gets what it has been starved of. The moment you start giving your body what it needs, you will automatically start getting rid of the surplus fat stored in your cells. Instead of starving yourself and having to struggle with stringent diet plans each and every day, you are finally about to turn the corner leading to your success.

You will get enough to eat and feel satisfied while regaining your natural well-proportioned body shape.

Raw Food and Body Temperature

"How can I keep warm in wintertime when I eat raw food?" This is a question often posed, especially from people who live in the colder climates of the north. You probably know the feeling of warmth on a cold winter day after consuming a large portion of hot soup or any other hot meal or drink. The same sensation can also be felt by drinking strong spirits, as they spread a feeling of warmth throughout your body. The reason for this kind of heat, although not quite simple, is the same in both instances.

If you had asked me years ago why we feel warm after eating hot food, I would have answered that the reason is obvious: the heat in the food heats our body. However, even though there is a direct transfer of heat from the food to our body, it is only minimal. The real reason for feeling warm is quite different.

Why Warm Food Makes You Feel Cold

When you eat heated or processed food, blood flow increases in your veins. White blood cells are redirected to your stomach in order to combat what you are eating because your body does not recognize what you are consuming as food. At the same time, your body's enzymes are overworked since the amount of enzymes in heated

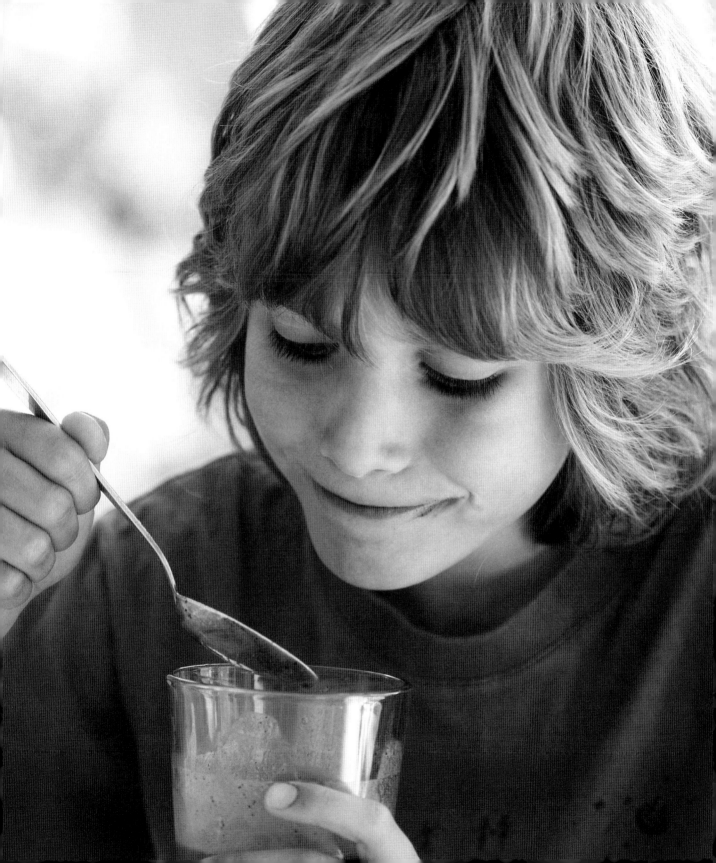

food is so much less than the amount found in raw food. Your body thus enters into defense mode, which is the cause of the warmth you experience.

Shortly after this initial warming effect, a secondary warming begins as a result of a chemical and biological process. When the heated food you have consumed enters your system, your adrenal glands are irritated. The adrenal glands, which are found just above the kidneys, start producing adrenaline and various other hormones. These hormones stimulate your sympathetic nervous system, which stimulates your state of alertness. The hormones also increase your heart rate and blood flow, again leading to the feeling of warmth that you experience.

But this feeling of warmth is short lived. After a brief time, your body becomes fatigued by the unnecessary additional work. Your heart needs a break, your nervous system weakens, and you start to feel tired and colder than you were before eating the heated food.

What often happens is that you remember the initial feeling of warmth and associate it with eating heated food. So you proceed to repeat this stimulation again and again, and this damaging routine wears down your body, especially the adrenal glands. Another undesired effect is that your resistance to cold diminishes with this process.

Yet another reason why eating warm food makes you feel cold is that warm food impedes your blood circulation. About 80 percent of your blood is found in the small blood vessels, known as capillaries, and only 20 percent flows in the larger arteries and veins. The miniscule capillaries get clogged up quickly by the large food particles from heated food, and your blood circulation becomes insufficient. This impeded circulation makes it more and more difficult for you to keep warm.

Why Raw Food Makes You Warm

Raw food regenerates your stamina and your adrenal glands, your central nervous system, and your heart, while at the same time helping to improve your blood circulation. All these factors contribute to your feeling nice and warm even on a cold winter's day.

If you feel cold during the first winter you eat raw food, this could be because your adrenal glands may be weakened. Your blood circulation is probably not functioning properly yet. Both effects may be due to years of sustained wear and tear. Most people will experience an improvement in their ability to regulate their body temperature after the first year of eating raw food. Until you feel this shift, wear more layers in the winter or try to increase your physical activity.

During the period when I ate meat and also when I switched to being a vegetarian and then a vegan, I used to be very sensitive to cold. When fall brought temperatures down to between 50–60 degrees Fahrenheit, I used to suffer from cold hands and feet.

Now, after becoming a raw foodist, I so enjoy an ice-cold dip in the sea, even when the water gets freezing cold in winter. I still enjoy the warmth from a fireplace, but cold does not affect me in the same way as before.

The Best Thing You Can Do for Earth

The Food and Agriculture Organization of the United Nations (FAO) published the report "Livestock's Long Shadow—Environmental Issues and Options" on November 29, 2006, in which the following was stated:

> "Livestock are one of the most significant contributors to today's most serious environmental problems. Urgent action is required to remedy the situation."

The meat industry consumes worrisome amounts of the Earth's resources. It generates 65 percent of the nitrous oxide, mostly from livestock manure, that is produced by human industry. These levels of nitrous oxide are 296 times the Global Warming Potential (GWP) of carbon dioxide and are the biggest contributor to deforestation and thus to the destruction of biodiversity and the extinction of species, polluting the Earth we live on and the air we breathe.

> "Nothing will benefit human health and increase chances of survival for life on Earth as much as the evolution to a vegetarian diet." (Albert Einstein).

By substituting part of your diet with raw food, you can help make the Earth a better place to live. You could start by buying more organic produce, by reducing your meat consumption, by buying fewer processed foods, or by becoming a vegetarian. Any of these choices will contribute positively to the environment.

Information in the following section is partly taken from the Food and Agriculture Organization of the United Nations and from EarthSave International and the World Wildlife Fund.

Clean Drinking Water for Everyone

Clean drinking water is a scarce resource in many places on Earth. Food production worldwide uses over 75 percent of all available freshwater. One of the main culprits is the meat production industry. Up to thirty-seven times more water is required to produce 2 pounds of meat than to produce 2 pounds of vegetables. This becomes a very substantial number at higher volumes; in the year 2000 the meat industry produced 514 billion pounds of meat, which translates to approximately 3,962 gallons of water used. We could reduce our water consumption dramatically by reducing the amount of meat we eat during a year.

Another way in which we can help ensure adequate supplies of clean drinking water is by eating organic produce. Pesticides used in the production of nonorganic farming seep into our groundwater and pollute it. In Denmark alone, over fifty types of pesticides have been found in the groundwater.

Simply stated: organic + raw food = more and cleaner drinking water.

Feed the Entire World's Population

The equivalent of 26 pounds of grain is required in order to produce 2 pounds of meat. In the United States alone, livestock production accounts for 70 percent of the grain consumed. Every year, Denmark imports 1.8 million tons of soy products used as animal feed.

The coefficient of utilization of land is several times better for planting crops than it is for rearing livestock. If these areas were used for growing fruit and vegetables instead, it would be possible to feed the entire world's population. Without increasing either the amount of arable land or the consumption of resources, we could eradicate world hunger if we switched over to a primarily vegetable-based diet.

Save Biodiversity

Since 2004, Brazil has been the world's largest exporter of beef—in all, sixty million head of cattle a year. In order to provide grazing land for all those cattle, huge areas of the Amazon jungle have been completely deforested— both legally and illegally. For every two pounds of meat produced in this area, twenty to thirty different types of trees and plants are destroyed, more than 1.3 tons of invaluable biomass in all. Over a hundred different types of insects, birds, small mammals, and reptiles are also killed.

If this development continues, it is estimated that seven million acres of rain forest in Brazil and Bolivia will disappear each year.

Reduce the Greenhouse Effect by 18 Percent

The world's livestock and other husbandry production contribute 18 percent to the total greenhouse effect and thus is the biggest single contributor to global warming. That is more than the entire transportation sector and almost as much as the entire greenhouse gas emissions of the United States. Sixty percent of Brazil's greenhouse gas emissions is directly or indirectly caused by deforestation and cattle farming. If the world's human population cut its meat consumption in half, we could reduce the emission of greenhouse gases by 9 percent.

Organic Farming Versus Pesticide Pollution

In 2000, Denmark, which has a population of only 5.5 million people, used 2,889 tons of pesticides and approximately 10,000 tons of chemical adjuvant. A total of about 13,000 tons of chemicals were spread on Danish fields. In the same year, 1,396 water-drilling sites, equal to 24 percent of examined drilling sites, were found to be contaminated by pesticides. And that is only in Denmark, where farmers are considered to be very effective at reducing the amounts of pollutants used in production.

Pesticides destroy local fauna and flora regardless of where they are used in the world. Over 90 percent of all insects, plants, and bacteria eradicated by pesticides are harmless or even beneficial to crops, to the environment, and to humans.

Organic farming does not make use of pesticides and thus does not contaminate local drinking water. You can play an influential part in reducing the amount of pesticides used in farming by eating more organic fruits and vegetables. This reduction is instrumental in maintaining a good supply of clean drinking water while ensuring that beneficial insects, plants, and bacteria are not exterminated.

Animal Welfare

In Denmark there are more pigs and cows than people. Pigs and cows are raised with the sole intent of ending up as meat as quickly as possible. The majority of these animals live under conditions that are unnatural to them and some of them are even directly mistreated.

There is no longer a need to kill animals. Nevertheless, the number of animals killed in the Danish meat industry is alarming. Humans are the only species that ruthlessly exploit other animals, resulting in billions of animals suffering and being killed every year.

Perhaps the biggest gift you can bestow on yourself and the rest of the thousands of animal species that inhabit this planet with you is to switch to a plant-based diet.

Protect the World's Oceans

Twenty-five percent of all fish caught in the world are bycatch (those caught unintentionally). In other words, one-fourth of all the fish caught are not the intended catch and are subsequently discarded. Enormous numbers of small fish, seals, birds, and even dolphins are killed, thrown out, or merely left to rot—with the few exceptions of when the bycatch is used to produce meat and bonemeal for animal feed.

The huge trawlers used by the fishing industry damage the seabed and kill everything in their way. Many fish have already gone extinct and many more have become endangered species, while the total fish population has been dramatically reduced in recent decades. Fish farms pollute both their fish and the surrounding waters with high concentrations of strong antibiotics and fish feces.

The seas are also being polluted by our overconsumption of packaging materials. The processed food industry uses huge amounts of packaging in producing frozen meals, soft drinks, and all manner of convenience foods. Some of this packaging ends up as ocean debris, along with so much of our other waste. There are huge garbage and debris fields floating around in our seas, known as "garbage patches."

Most of us don't realize how many industries contribute to the pollution of our waterways. In the United States, cattle farming produces 219 billion gallons of manure each year, manure that seeps into our rivers and groundwater. Almost 80 percent of that manure ends up in the Mississippi River, which flows into the Gulf of Mexico, leaving a wasteland in its wake.

It does not take a Herculean effort to save the world's oceans. You can choose to either reduce your consumption of meat, fish, and processed foods or change your diet to more plant-based and raw food. Regardless of what you choose, the above examples show how even small changes carry the potential for great improvements.

Save on Electricity

The food industry today uses enormous amounts of energy on processing foods and on producing artificial additives. There are factory buildings full of chickens and stables choked with cattle. Factories as well as stables need to be heated. Supermarkets need huge freezers; and when consumers bring home their food, they use a refrigerator, a stove, a toaster, and a microwave oven to store and prepare their food.

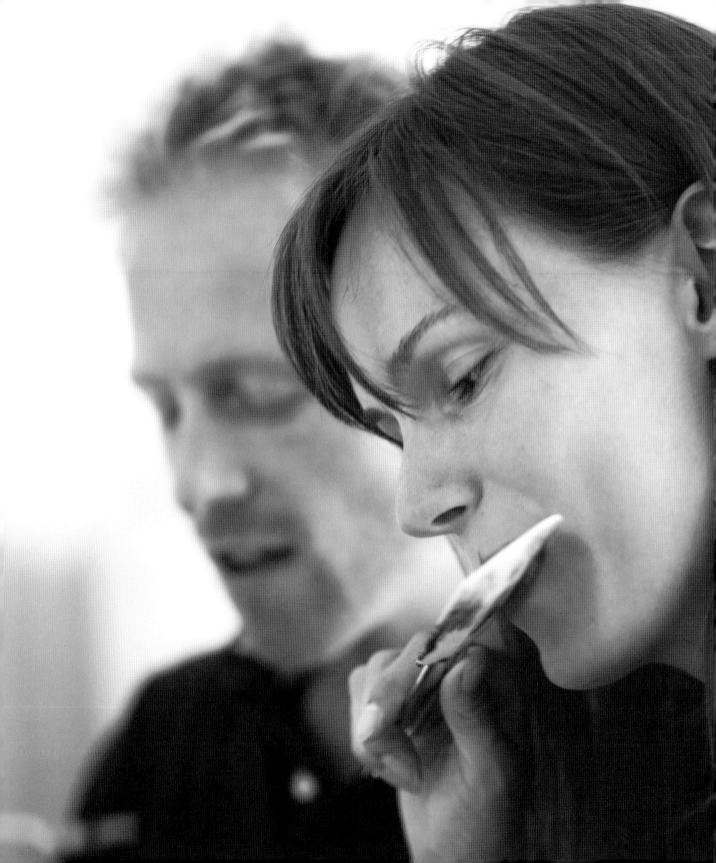

All this amounts to a huge consumption of energy that can be reduced as you switch to eating more raw food.

Conclusion

As a consumer, you have a great deal of power, perhaps more than you are aware of. By exercising your freedom of choice each and every day in the way you choose to live and in your buying habits, you can make a significant difference without having to compromise your standard of living. Your contributions can help increase the supply of clean drinking water, eradicate famine, reduce the emissions of greenhouse gases, secure biodiversity, save the seas, minimize pollution, and reduce the suffering of animals.

This is not about being self-righteous or fanatical. It is not about giving up progress and all that is good—on the contrary. It is about being more thankful for what we have, appreciating it, and treating it with consideration—not because we have to, but because it is simply the best we can do for ourselves, and for life on Earth.

With raw food you can make a difference to the world's health while improving your own.

Why We Prefer Raw Food

Jens's Story

Do you want your food raw or heated?

This is probably not a question you are used to asking yourself. Actually, the majority of the people to whom I have introduced raw food had never really considered their food preparation choices. Why should they question something that seems so natural? If you had asked me the question a couple of years back my answer would have invariably been: hot food, please. Why would I have wanted to eat raw food? I liked the taste of the food I ate and I considered my lifestyle to be reasonably healthy.

I was fine and healthy. Admittedly, I could no longer party for three nights in a row and with little or no sleep still be able to show up for work full of energy. But that was not so important for me any longer. When I looked at my friends and people I knew, I was still the one with the most energy—the one who, even though he had taught a seminar from 8 a.m. to 11 p.m. three days in a row, got up at 6 a.m. to do yoga, run on the beach, or go for a dip in the freezing cold sea.

Still, I was not in as good shape as before. I had some difficulty running long distance and fast due to a couple of pulled muscles in my thigh and a bit of a problem with one of my knees. My fitness rating was way above average and my body fat percentage was only 10 but my body needed longer to recuperate.

I was told that it was totally normal to not have the energy I wanted to have; that I was just experiencing the normal signs of aging, and we all lose energy as we grow older. I was, after all, not eighteen any longer; I was in my thirties.

Frankly, that was just not enough for me. I wanted to live an extraordinary life, not settle for second best. I wanted to be able to pursue my dreams without being held back by my body. I wanted to be happier and healthier each day that went by. I also wanted it to be possible for others to follow suit. A new motto entered my mind and lodged there: "May your wildest dreams and aspirations become the footsteps that you leave in the sand tomorrow."

I wanted to be just as vital and alive as I had been before, and hopefully even more so. I wanted to gush energy and vitality. I wanted to be able to give the best to the people I helped so they too could live a life that surpassed their own dreams. That is why I became interested in raw food and now give a different answer to the question of whether I want my food hot or not.

Why did I change my mind?

I freely admit that I have read numerous articles and books on nutrition, health, and longevity. I have attended lectures and seminars, but that is not the real reason why I prefer going 100 percent raw. It aroused my curiosity and captured my interest, but the reason was so much simpler:

I tried raw food!

For a period I ate raw food, then stopped. I started again and stopped. I tried eating 100 percent raw and then 50 percent raw. I tried combining raw food with heated food and even sometimes ate as I had done earlier—not because it was any kind of personal test or experiment, but because I had an insatiable craving for the kind of food that I had been accustomed to. Other times it was just an old habit I fell back on, reverting to cruise control and not being totally aware of what I was doing. However, I realized that when I ate food that was heated or in any other fashion processed, it just did not give me the satisfaction I wanted.

The more I got in touch with my own needs, the greater the consequences. Food I had earlier relished eating now made me tired, restless, lethargic, or hyperactive, as if I had been taking drugs or had swallowed a handful of sleeping pills. It influenced my mood and I felt as if my stomach had been filled with concrete.

I experienced the opposite feeling during the periods when I ate raw food. I experienced an inner peace and a feeling of finding my inner equilibrium. My need to overeat or eat for comfort had completely disappeared. I had more energy and *joie de vivre.* I became more resilient. My skin was clearer and had that radiant sun-kissed look. I needed less sleep and felt like a cloud had been lifted from my mind. My senses became sharper: everything seemed to taste and smell better. My attention span increased and I found it very easy to live in the moment. I became very keen on sensing my own needs and satisfying them, while feeling able to give more to those around me. It seemed as if by magic everything in life became better. I felt liberated, happy, and strong.

As I switched back and forth between raw food and heated food, I became more and more impressed by the wonderful advantages of eating raw food. Today, I will not eat anything else.

For me, eating raw food feels like the ultimate luxury. It tastes heavenly and I feel completely satisfied after each and every meal, all day long. That I have become better looking, healthier, and happier is just a wonderful addition.

So why do I prefer raw food?

Besides falling in love and becoming a father, it is the change that has most greatly improved my quality of life.

Vibeke's Story

The first time I heard about raw food I was totally fascinated by what it could do for our bodies and minds, fascinated by what it could do for our world and the state of the Earth. I first heard about raw food at a course I attended in the United States. As I listened to David Wolfe, a raw food expert, I was especially enchanted by the positive influence raw food could have on our health and consciousness.

"The cleaner you eat, the clearer you see." (David Wolfe)

I subsequently bought lots of books on raw food but quickly found out that the books available on the market had a very exotic approach to recipes, and it was not easy to acquire all the necessary ingredients in Denmark.

So even though I really wanted to change my diet to raw food it was not feasible. It was only when I met Jens, who taught me his own style of preparing delicious and easy dishes, that my transition to raw food truly began.

Jens gave me recipes that were easy to follow and showed me how to make food that tasted heavenly.

The quantum leap improvement I experienced in my quality of life after such a short period of eating raw food was something I had to share with the entire world. I experienced a heightened state of awareness, intuition, vitality, flow of ideas, and health. I have never discovered anything that is so simple, yet can have such a huge impact. It is indescribable. I want to show what raw food is so that every one of you who may want to try it can experience what it means to eat raw.

How I Started Eating Raw Food   It can be done very simply. If you are curious, my advice is to take it one step at a time. I started by removing everything in my kitchen that was not raw food, and began experimenting with raw breakfasts, smoothies, and salads. I quickly got the hang of the basic elements and things just took off from there. The more I ate raw food, the more I craved it. Today, I feel best when I eat 100 percent raw food.

What Raw Food Has Meant for Me   Raw food has had a profound impact on my physical health and sense of well-being. I feel healthier and stronger than ever before. My body is more supple, my skin is more radiant, and my nails are stronger. I no longer suffer from joint and muscle pains, and I have gotten rid of various forms of allergies. I used to be allergic to nickel, grass, birch, and mugwort, and suffered from pollen allergies as early in the year as February. Because of my nickel allergy, I could not eat several types of nuts and fruits, but now after going raw, I can indulge all I want. All these ailments have been alleviated by a raw food diet. Perhaps the best part of it is that I have not had one sick day since I changed my diet over to raw food.

Raw food has also given me a huge boost of *joie de vivre* and a greatly improved quality of life. Raw food cleanses and heals. I feel my senses are more open and that a filter has been removed so I see everything more clearly than before. My intuition for what is good or bad for me has been restored. Creativity and ideas fill me in a way I had never experienced before.

I have also regained my enjoyment of food again, and the desire to prepare it. For years I had not really enjoyed food. I had eaten a reasonably healthy and organic diet but the food just did not taste of much. Raw food has given me a fantastic gourmet sense. It is like having love flow down your throat. I hope you will have the same experience.

To go raw is very simple. It feels natural. Moreover, it is one of the most sustainable ways of living in harmony with nature.

I am very grateful for all that raw food has contributed to in my life—and grateful that Jens was convinced to write this book.

Enjoy it! It is fantastic! Unsurpassed!

Quality Products and the Presence of Love

The most important factor in achieving success with raw food is using good quality, fresh, organic, seasonal produce. Quality is the surest way to delicious food in any kitchen. Why is that so?

Quality produce tastes better, smells better, is more nuanced, and offers a variety of color—all aspects necessary for a well-prepared meal. Raw food offers lush and seductive tastes, mouthwatering smells, irresistible and alluring beauty to beguile your eyes: food that you just can't resist tasting.

I was very privileged to grow up in a home with a garden. My father, who grew up on a fruit orchard, taught me at a very early age that there is a huge difference between apples left to naturally ripen on the tree in our garden—plucked just as they reached their full potential for taste and quality—and apples that are bought, cooled, sprayed, and flown in from overseas. I had never heard of organic farming then; I just instinctively knew the apples tasted better.

My childhood was also blessed with a mother who prepared solid Danish dishes with local, seasonal vegetables and always served them with an abundance of fresh salad. In spring, she would serve ground beef with new Danish onions and potatoes and in winter we would have meatballs with creamy cooked cabbage. The spices my mother used were salt, pepper, chives, and parsley. Simple yet delicious, with every meal prepared from scratch. Basic ingredients are still very important to me—ingredients packed with taste and vitality and served in their simplest form.

No one specific recipe or preparation method is the right one; our tastes can vary from dish to dish depending on personal preference. But one thing is for sure: presence, attention to details, making adjustments where necessary, and love all contribute to creating the sublime experience of pleasure derived from great-tasting food. Taste your food as you prepare it; sometimes all that is needed is a slight adjustment to bring a dish up to the level of sublime taste.

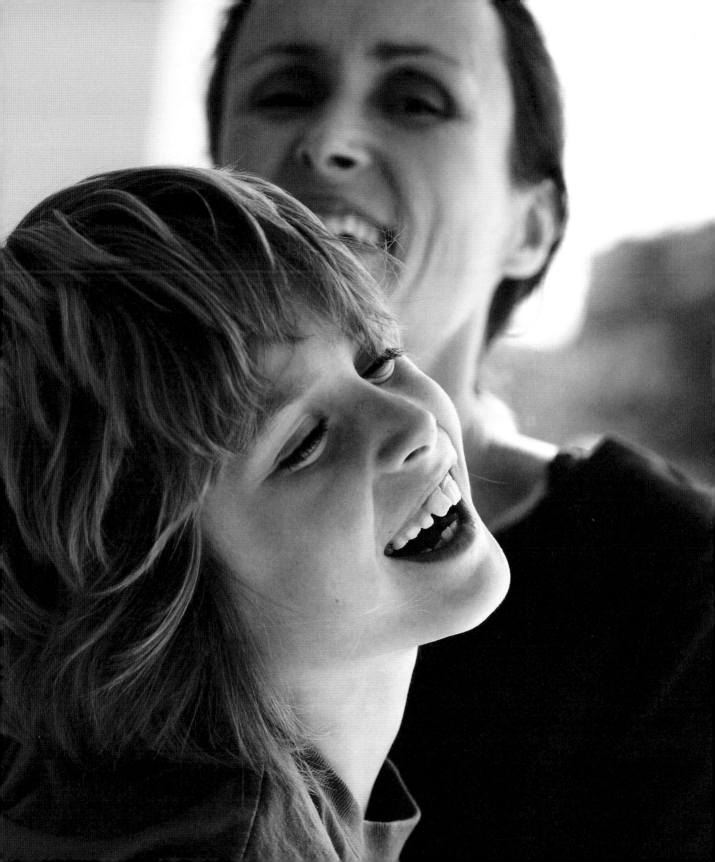

Eating Organic

Whenever I am asked why we should eat organic, I give this answer: No one can decide on your behalf if you should eat organic food, but the next time you have a choice between an organic product and a conventional one, ask yourself the following question: Do I feel like drinking a small glass of pesticide?

Or how about drinking a teaspoon of fertilizer, thickening powder, thinning powder, or bleach?

You wouldn't like that, would you?

I know for sure I wouldn't. And the idea of serving such things to my daughter or friends is, frankly, unthinkable. What and how you like to eat is really none of my business, but when I am the cook, I am adamant in my choice of organic ingredients.

It is impossible to wash pesticides off your food. Vegetables, fruits, and all the rest of the food we eat are living organisms that absorb nutrients from other substances they contact through their roots and external shell or peel. This means that pesticides are absorbed into the structure of the vegetables or fruits that you eat.

In 2000, about 13,000 tons of chemicals, in the form of pesticides and other toxins, were spread over the fields of Denmark. The year before that, it was found that 33 percent of Danish fruit and 62 percent of imported fruit was contaminated with pesticides; for vegetables the number amounted to 6 percent for homegrown vegetables and 22 percent for imported ones.

Generally speaking, all pesticides and processing methods are intended to kill life. Killing life that once was food can result in showcase products that can be kept looking fresh and lush for long periods of time—some seemingly forever. This process is reminiscent of the embalming processes practiced by the ancient Egyptians. But we are not dead yet, are we?

The best route to beauty is to keep the cells in your body alive. Everything dead decomposes, while everything alive regenerates. I readily admit that I want to look good, so for me organic equals beauty. Sometimes vanity is fantastic!

Even though the majority of us eat food because it tastes good, we also want it to be full of nutritious energy. We want to have a physique that enables us to do whatever we want—whether it be climbing Mount Everest, dancing all night long, walking for hours sightseeing in New York or Tokyo, laughing and tumbling about with our children and grandchildren, or having fantastic sex for hours with our partner ...

For me personally, organic is not a matter of choice; it is a must. Nonorganic products are only a last resort, something I would rather live without.

My partner, Naja, loves cashew nuts and eats lots of them. But that has not always been the case. She used to have allergic reactions after eating just a couple of nuts. However, when we switched over to buying only organic cashews, her discomfort disappeared almost overnight.

Vibeke used to have the same problem when eating almonds. If she ate just one nut, she would get an itching and irritating sensation in her throat. When she switched to organic almonds, she suddenly discovered that she could eat as many as she liked without any discomfort at all.

Do you experience any uncomfortable reactions when eating nuts? Or have you been told that you are allergic or have an intolerance? It is very possible that you can eat these nuts as long as they are organically produced. It is of course not certain that this applies to you, so perhaps you should start with a very small amount of organic nuts and feel your way forward.

Enjoyment and Health

Have you ever wondered why the French and the Italians can eat huge amounts of white bread and pasta and eat late at night, yet still seem to be healthy? They usually eat dinner at around 10 p.m. and their breakfast often consists of only coffee and a croissant or cookie. What is more, they pour lots of olive oil on everything they eat. We in northern Europe are constantly reminded that these habits are unhealthy. How do they manage, then? What is their secret?

I think it boils down to the simple fact that the French and Italians are passionate about food—they truly enjoy eating. For them, eating is a social encounter with family and friends and they set aside time to enjoy it. Do like the Italians do: eat when you eat. Give yourself time to be present in the moment. Turn off the TV and radio, hide away your newspaper, and keep that book for later. Take the time to prepare tempting and appetizing food and enjoy eating it together with others. Prepare food together, laugh, relax, and give yourself time to enjoy life.

There are several physical and psychological factors that contribute to the fact that enjoying your food is healthy, but you do not need to learn about the scientific experiments and studies. Just listen to your body, eat, and be happy!

Animal Protein and Human Illnesses

Protein consists of long chains of amino acids that constitute vital components for a healthy body. Your body most needed proteins when you were a newborn baby. However, breast milk, which was sufficient for you to grow strong and healthy, contains less than 2 percent protein. Several years later, as an adult, your body has stopped growing, but you still need to replenish the supplies of amino acids used by your body. You get these proteins through the food you eat. However, it matters a great deal what source you get your proteins from, as you will see from the following research results.

Dr. T. Colin Campbell, who headed one of the most ambitious research projects on nutrition and health, the China Study, which was conducted in collaboration with Oxford University, Cornell University, and the Chinese Academy of Preventive Medicine, made the following remarks:

> "People who eat large amounts of animal products suffer most from chronic ailments. Even small amounts of animal-based substances in your diet can have adverse effects. Cancer, cardiovascular disorders, diabetes, obesity, all ailments that we suffer from in our modern society, can actually be prevented and treated by consuming a diet of organically produced vegetables."

For almost fifty years, Dr. Campbell has designed and directed large research projects in the areas of nutrition and health. He has given speeches to the U.S. Congress and to many public agencies. He is author or coauthor of more than 350 scientific articles. He has appeared on over twenty-five TV shows and has been featured in lead stories in the *New York Times* and *USA Today*. His research projects are supported by the National Institutes of Health, the American Cancer Society, and the American Institute for Cancer Research, so his statements should be taken seriously.

Based on their results, the China Study group recommended that we get our proteins from plant-based foods, as these are the healthiest and most beneficial. Plant-based proteins enable a slower and more stable buildup of protein in your body. The United States Department of Agriculture (USDA) has stated that the daily protein requirement can easily be met through eating vegetables.

Dark green vegetables such as spinach, broccoli, and kale include large amounts of protein, as do nuts, seeds, and legumes. (If you eat raw food, remember to soak legumes and wait till they sprout, as this will ensure optimal nutritional value.) Regardless of how you choose to proceed, you will most assuredly be able to get the required amount of proteins through a varied vegetable diet.

Vitamin B12

Even though on a raw food diet you will most likely feel better than ever before, one thing that is crucial to keep in mind when you follow such a regime is to ensure that you are getting sufficient amounts of vitamin B12.

Vitamins are formed by bacteria that live in water, in soil, and in the digestive system of animals and humans. However, because bacteria live in the large intestinal tract and your body absorbs vitamin B12 through your small intestine, it is not possible to absorb the vitamin. In prehistoric times, humans ingested their vitamin B12 through the soil on their vegetables. But today, with all our vegetables being rigorously washed, the risk for suffering from a vitamin B12 deficiency is very high.

If you eat a vegan diet or restrict yourself to raw food for long periods, you will need to ensure that you take a B12 supplement; even though you only need minute amounts, it is essential. Make sure that the supplement includes an active form of B12 such as adenosylcobalamin, methylcobalamin, cyanocobalamin, or hydroxocobalamin.

Essential Minerals

Minerals are essential building blocks in all your body's organs and cellular structures. In a way, your body is constructed of minerals. Moreover, minerals are responsible for activating vitamins and enzyme components in your body. In the absence of essential minerals and trace minerals, you would not be able to survive.

Minerals must be miniscule for your body to absorb them, for the minerals to enter into your cells where they are needed. They cannot exceed one-millionth of a meter, also known as the angstrom size. If minerals are larger, they can potentially turn into toxic accumulations in various parts of your body.

> "Ultimately you can trace each and every illness, every discomfort and every disease back to a mineral deficiency." (Dr. Linus Pauling, two-time Nobel laureate).

One of the reasons why organic fruits and vegetables are good for you is that they contain large amounts of minerals that your body can easily absorb and use for vital functions that keep you healthy and happy. Besides fruits and vegetables, various types of seaweed provide easy-to-absorb minerals and trace minerals. Kelp and dulse, both dried seaweeds, are healthy alternatives to salt. They include loads of essential minerals and trace minerals, such as iodine. They are also a good taste-enhancer for your food. Sodium chloride, better known as table salt, is not a good source of minerals. It has no nutritional value and is even harmful to your body. If you choose to use salt, remember to use it sparingly and to choose the best available quality. The best types are unrefined sea salt or Himalayan salt, while the worst types are the cheap, ordinary table salts.

Water and Fluids

Fluid deficiency, or dehydration, is the most common cause of fatigue during the day. Often the signs that you may construe as hunger are in fact signs that you are thirsty. If you wait to drink until you start feeling thirsty, you are already dehydrated. When your cells start to dehydrate they start to die.

In 2001, a study was conducted among the British participants in the Olympic Games. It showed that a 1 percent fluid deficiency led to a loss of performance equaling 5 percent. This is not only important for top athletes. Your entire metabolic system and your brain will shut down when you reach a state of dehydration. Your skin dries out and loses its elasticity and you age faster.

Some years ago there was a widespread campaign with the slogan "You are what you eat." When you consider that your body consists of more than 70 percent water, shouldn't your diet then include at least as much water?

All that you eat must be transformed into fluid in order to be absorbed by your body. When you fry, cook, or bake food, the ingredients' natural water content evaporates. So not only does digesting cooked food not replenish your body's vital need for fluids, it also drains your body of its water reserves.

When you eat raw food, your body does not need extra water to initiate the digestion process. All raw vegetables and fruits are water-saturated, with some of them containing 90 percent water. When you eat raw food, you will not become easily dehydrated as your diet provides you with a sufficient amount of water.

One of the reasons why certain berries, fruits, and vegetables (such as beetroots or blueberries) leave stains is that they are wetter than other vegetables or fruits. "Wetter" here means that the surface tension in their juices is low. This is the reason why different substances in the juice, such as the color, easily penetrate the fibers in your fine summer tablecloth, on which your child accidentally put a handful of ripe berries. This property in berries is highly beneficial for you. It is not only the coloring agent that enters your body and your cells—all the nutrients do the same.

To sum up: raw food has a much higher level of fluids than heated food and also includes vital nutrients. Since the fluid found in vegetables and fruits has a low surface tension, nutrients can flow unhindered into your body and lodge exactly where you need them most.

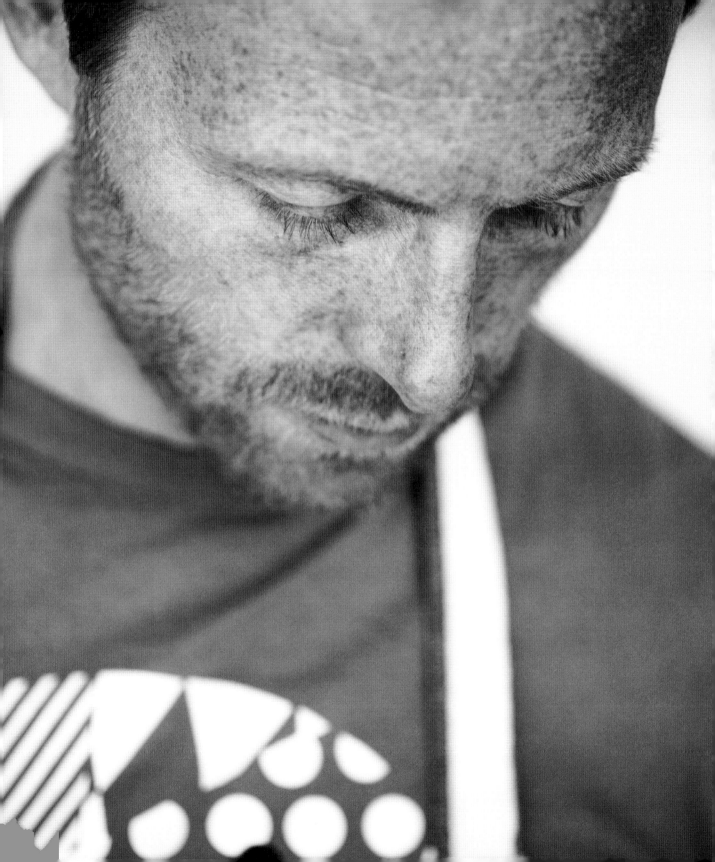

What About Sugar?

There are many ways of sweetening with raw food. You can use sweet fresh fruits such as bananas, dry fruits, stevia, or various forms of agave. The taste and consistency differ with these ingredients, and some methods of sweetening are better for some dishes than others. It is also important to note that the speed at which a sweetener is absorbed in your body depends on the type used. This is perhaps the reason why I especially covet certain types of agave nectar and stevia, as these enable you to maintain a stable blood sugar level.

As you enjoy the various cakes, desserts, and smoothies in this book, you will find that they are just as sweet in taste as those using conventional sugars; but unlike ordinary sweeteners, all these delicious raw food temptations are healthy and good for you. By using healthy sweeteners, you ensure that your dishes are packed with useful vitamins, enzymes, and other essential nutrients. And it will be easier for you to transition to a raw diet.

It is wonderful at long last to be able to enjoy a cookbook packed with recipes for delicious desserts that you can enjoy with a good conscience, knowing that you are actually doing good for your body by eating them!

How to Use This Book

Discover Your Own Cooking Style

There are many ways to enjoy this book. You can use it to discover favorite new recipes and serve them with the foods you normally eat. You can find inspiration from the dishes and play around a bit with the raw food concept. You could substitute one daily meal with raw food or you could go raw 80 percent or 100 percent of the time. You can enjoy a brief flirtation with raw food or launch into a passionate desire to change your lifestyle. What you choose is entirely up to you.

When first introduced to the concept of raw food, I had no intention of going 100 percent raw. Now that I have truly experienced the wonders of going raw, however, I will not eat anything else.

The book does not specify how many servings each recipe yields. That was done on purpose, as a way of giving you the freedom to do as you please—serve the dishes on their own or as side dishes, serve them buffet style, or just as a quick snack.

Be creative and come up with your own fantastic versions of the dishes. The fact that there are no recommended serving portions enhances your awareness that you should feel your way to what works best for you.

How much a person can eat is very individual, not just to them but to their mood or circumstances. Sometimes I can eat four helpings at one sitting; at other times I don't feel like or need such large portions.

Adjust the recipes to suit your needs. Some oranges are sour, others are small, some have a robust taste while others are more delicate. Some days your body craves more greens, other days more oil. Sometimes you may feel a need to add lots of spices, while other days you just want to taste the unadulterated, clean taste of raw ingredients.

Look at, touch, and taste the food as you prepare it and eat it. Get a feel for how it should be: drier, oilier, crisp, sweet, or sour. Take your time to consider the possibilities for both preparation style and quantities; whether you can suffice with half a portion or if you should double up on all the ingredients.

Preparing food is about love, nourishment, and enjoyment. So feel your way forward like you are newly in love: taste it, play with it, and let it beguile you.

Experiment and Substitute

Even though this book is packed with complete recipes, it is my hope that you will also be inspired to experiment in your own way with raw food. Whether you choose to follow the recipes point by point or just seek inspiration for your own experiments, it is worth noting that all the recipes can easily be adjusted and modified.

Let's say you don't have hazelnuts in your kitchen cabinet. No worries; just use any other nuts you have. You could even use sunflower seeds as a substitute for nuts in some of the recipes. Almost any ingredient can be substituted with something else. If you have difficulty finding some of the nuts, or you perhaps don't like them or just don't feel like eating them on a given day, substitute something else.

Of course dates are different from figs and raisins, just as hazelnuts are different from cashews, both in taste and texture. The same applies to baby spinach, arugula, and iceberg lettuce. But those differences enable you to modify a dish to suit your palate or use ingredients that you have on hand at home. You will quickly establish your favorites, and these may change over a period of time. There will inevitably be various combinations of ingredients that you like better than others; you may find that carrots are more suitable for pasta than squash or vice versa.

Try experimenting and substitute with what you already have in your kitchen.

Recipes

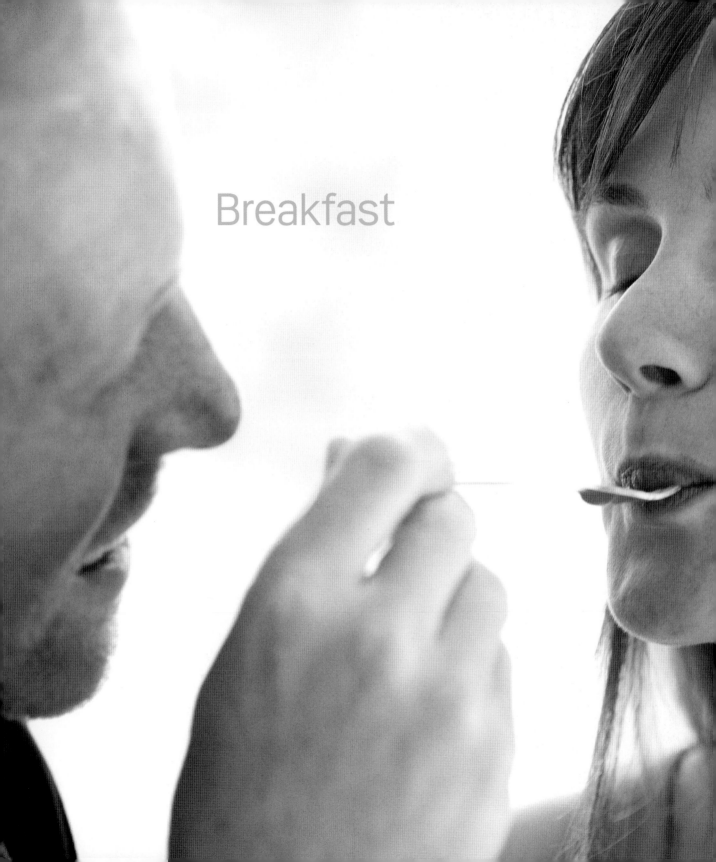

Breakfast

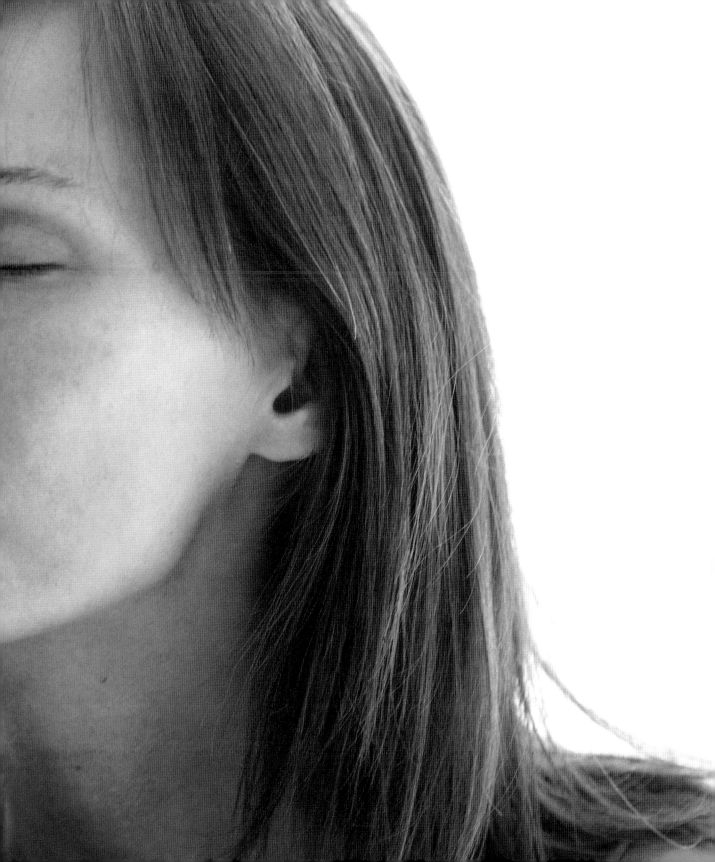

Cabbage Slaw with Cacao

Cabbage slaw (p. 134)
Raw cacao
Cacao pieces or nibs (optional)

Mix the cacao with the slaw.

This will give you a very healthy, fiber-rich breakfast with a taste of cacao.

For me, it is like having Cocoa Krispies for breakfast, without the sugar and the additives.

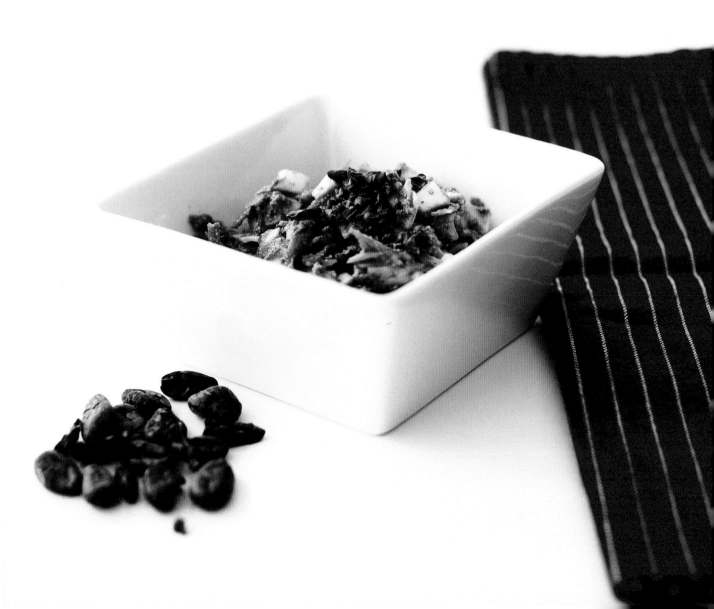

Delicious Buckwheat Porridge

2 cups (5 deciliters) buckwheat, soaked for 6 hours and sprouted 1–2 days
1 apple, cored
6 dates, pitted
½ tablespoon cinnamon
½ teaspoon vanilla
1 pinch of salt
½ cup (1 dl) raisins
1 sliced banana

Soak the buckwheat in water for 6 hours, then drain. Allow it to sprout for 1–2 days in a bowl covered with a dish-towel; rinse the sprouts two or three times a day.

Mix buckwheat, apple, dates, cinnamon, and vanilla in a food processor and blend until it has the desired consistency. Season with salt and mix in the raisins and banana slices.

Serve with a couple of thinly sliced apples and a sprinkle of cinnamon.

When I started eating raw food, this quickly became my favorite breakfast.

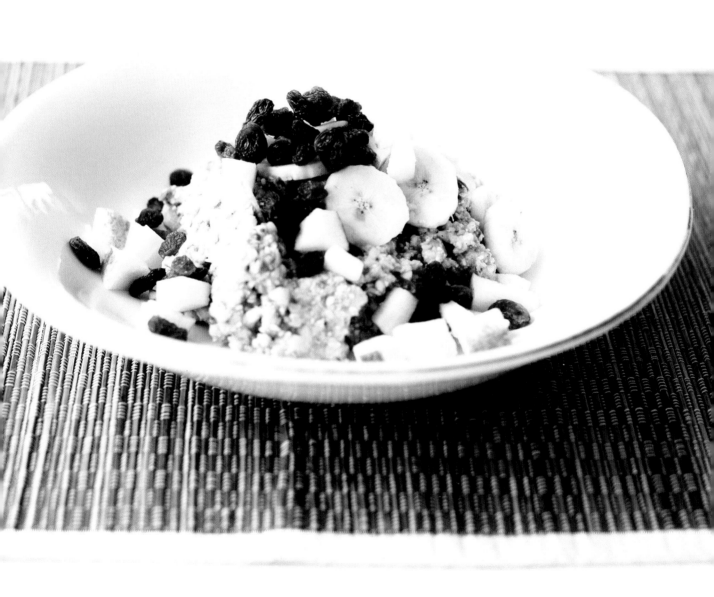

Morning Salad

2 pears
1 banana
½ cup (1 dl) almonds, soaked overnight and coarsely chopped
4 dates, pitted
1 tablespoon cacao bits
1 teaspoon grated ginger
1 tablespoon crushed linseed
½ teaspoon cinnamon

Cut pears, banana, and dates into appropriate portions and mix with the other ingredients.

Try serving the salad with cold rooibos nut milk (p. 272) or almond milk (p. 270).

You can also add buckwheat or quinoa soaked for at least 24 hours.

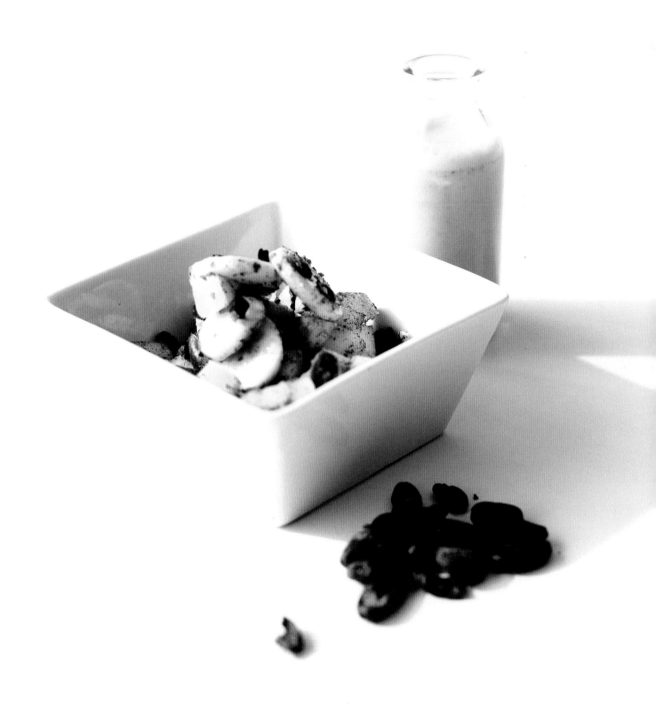

Fruit Salad

1 banana
5 strawberries
1 apple
¼ melon
1 orange
½ cup (1 dl) hazelnuts, coarsely chopped
2 tablespoons cacao bits

Cut the fruit into desired sizes and put it in a bowl. Mix with nuts and cacao.

If you feel like indulging yourself, you can add some heavenly vanilla cream to the salad (p. 262).

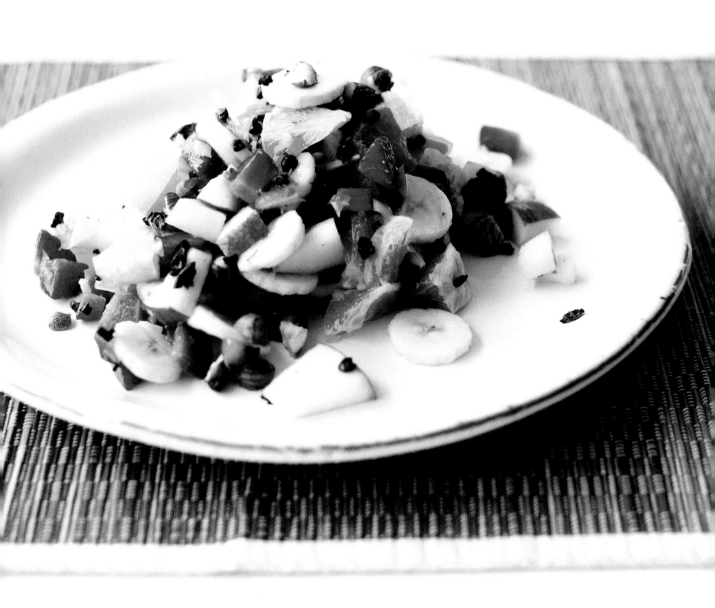

Raw Yogurt

2½ cups (6 dls) nuts or seeds, soaked
1¼ cups (3 dls) water

Soak cashews, macadamia nuts, almonds, or sunflower seeds in plenty of water overnight. Throw water out after soaking. If you use almonds, remove the skins before using them.

Mix nuts and water in a blender. Pour the thick milk through a nut-milk bag or a dishtowel. If you like, you can save the nut meat and use it in an other dish.

Leave the milk at room temperature for 8–12 hours covered with a dishtowel. The milk will begin to separate.

Refrigerate for at least 8–12 hours so the yogurt on top will have time to accumulate and stiffen.

Carefully pour the mix into a container with a spoon without disturbing the fluid at the bottom. The yogurt can stay fresh for 5 days in the refrigerator.

For a yogurt flavor, serve with berries and agave nectar.

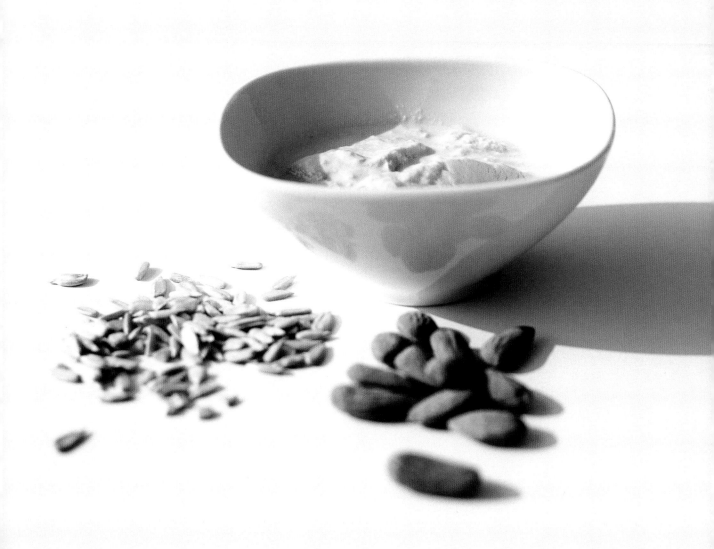

Muesli

¾ cup (2 dls) nuts, coarsely chopped
¼ cup (½ dl) sunflower seeds
½ cup (1 dl) blueberries or raspberries
½ cup (1 dl) apple, diced
½ cup (1 dl) dried figs, diced
Coconut

Mix the ingredients in a bowl and sprinkle with coconut.

Serve with your favorite nut milk (p. 269).

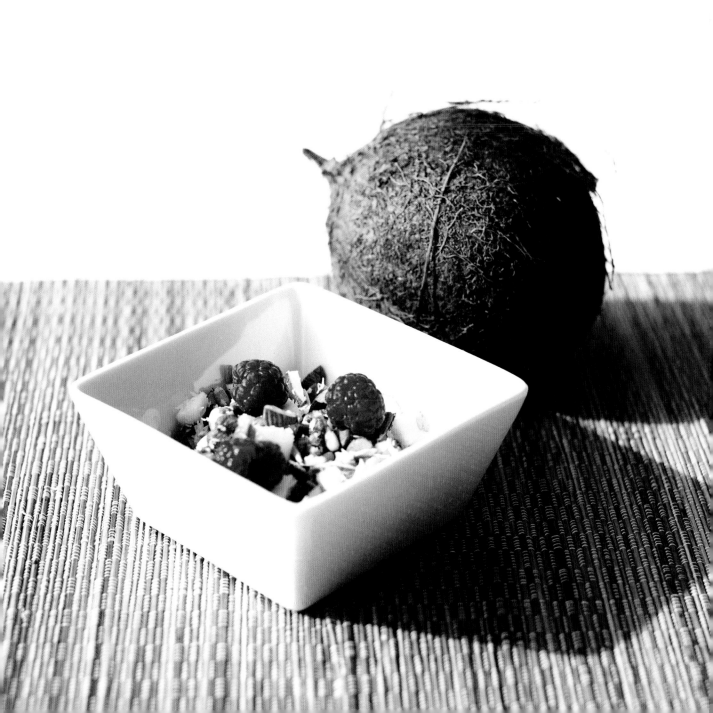

Yummy Oat Porridge

2 cups (5 dls) oatmeal, soaked for 1–3 days (change water and rinse at least once a day)*
½ cup (1 dl) dates, pitted
½ tablespoon cinnamon
1 pinch of salt
¾ cup (2 dls) raisins

Drain oatmeal and pour into a food processor, add dates and cinnamon, and blend to the desired consistency. Season with salt and mix in the raisins.

Serve as is or add extra fruit such as sliced kiwi or strawberries.

If the dates are too dry, it is a good idea to soak them for a few hours before use. (You can keep the soak water to use as a sweetener in a smoothie.)

You can vary the taste by adding almonds (soaked overnight) or coconut flour.

*Soaking the oatmeal makes it easier for your body to digest the porridge and thus absorb the nutrients.

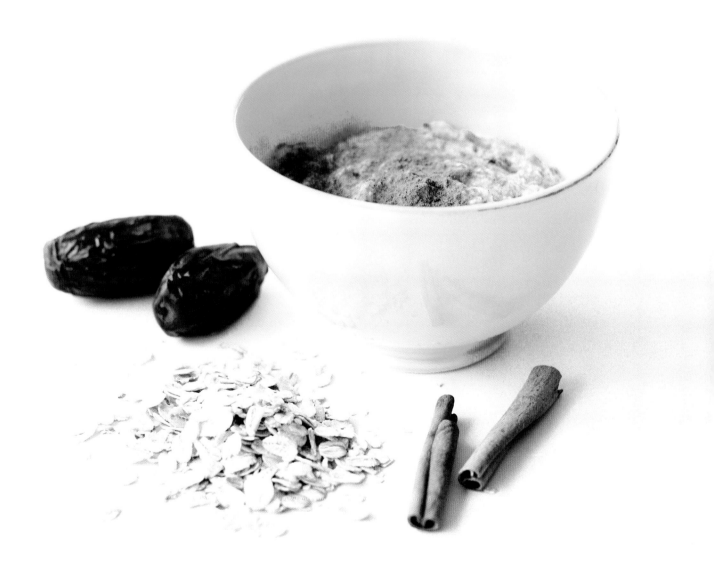

Fruit Plate

1 banana
1 kiwi
1 slice of watermelon
1 orange
2–3 dried dates
1 handful of nuts

Arrange the fresh fruit on a plate and enjoy their wonderful colors and aromas.

Use any combination of seasonal fruit, combining different colors but keeping it simple. Here is ample opportunity to experiment.

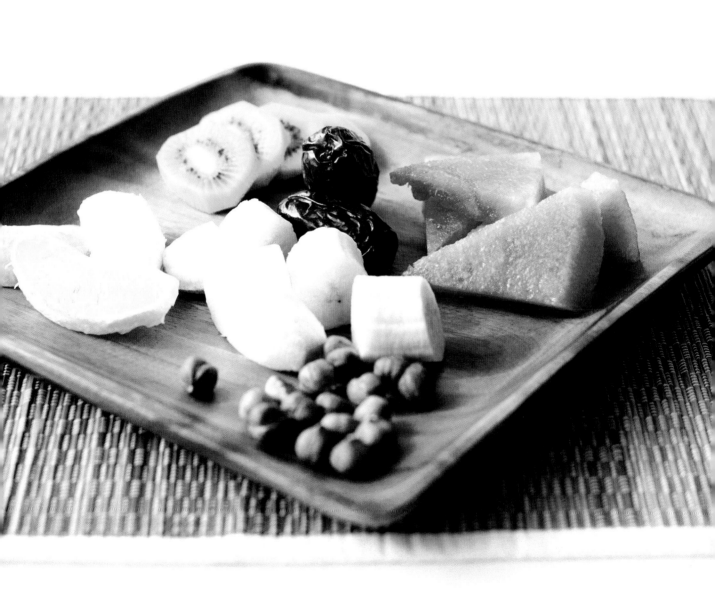

Look-alike Scrambled Eggs with Bacon

3 ears of corn or 10.5 ounces (300g) frozen corn
¼ head of cauliflower
1 shallot
¼ cup (½ dl) cold-pressed grapeseed oil
1 small bunch of parsley or chives
1 red bell pepper
Salt and pepper
1 clove garlic, minced
1 handful of sun-dried tomatoes ("bacon")

2 tablespoons olive oil or other oil of your choice
1 teaspoon herbal salt
Cherry tomato

Cut the kernels off the cobs (or thaw the frozen corn). Pour half of the kernels into a food processor with the cauliflower, shallots, garlic, and oil. Dice the red bell pepper and chop the parsley or chives. Mix it all in a bowl and season with salt and pepper.

Cut the sun-dried tomatoes into slices and put them in a bag. Pour the oil and salt into the bag, seal, and shake.

Arrange the "scrambled eggs" on a plate with the "bacon" and garnish with a little parsley and a cherry tomato.

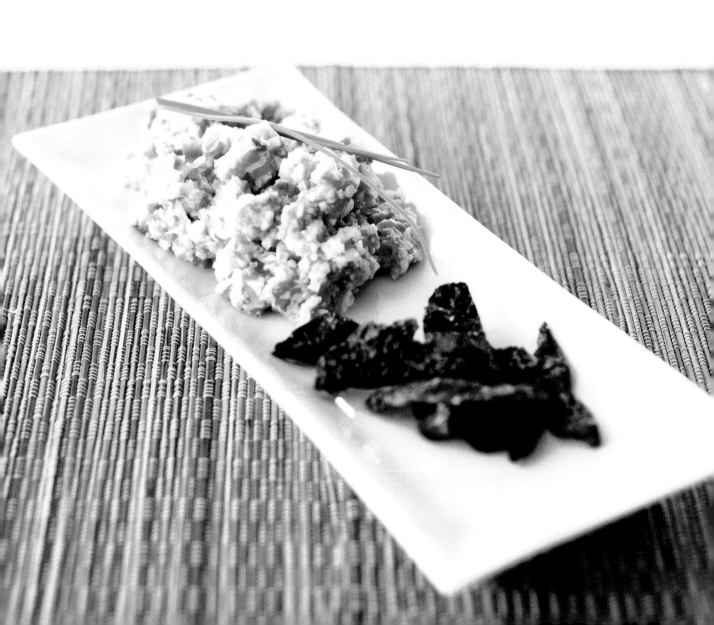

Fake Baked Beans in Tomato Sauce

1¾ cups (4 dls) barley or spelt, soaked for 6 hours
2 tomatoes
3 tablespoons agave nectar
1 teaspoon apple cider vinegar
Salt and pepper
4 sun-dried tomatoes, sliced

Soak the barley for 6 hours, drain, and let sprout for 1–2 days in a bowl covered with a dishtowel, rinsing two or three times a day until germinated.

Prepare the tomato sauce by cutting the fresh tomatoes into quarters. Remove the seeds and tomato juice. Pour into a blender with the other ingredients and blend until the sauce is smooth.

Mix the tomato sauce and barley in a bowl and allow the mixture to soak for a few hours so the flavor of the sauce blends into the grain.

Serve with the sliced sun-dried tomatoes. They make a fine "bacon," just healthier.

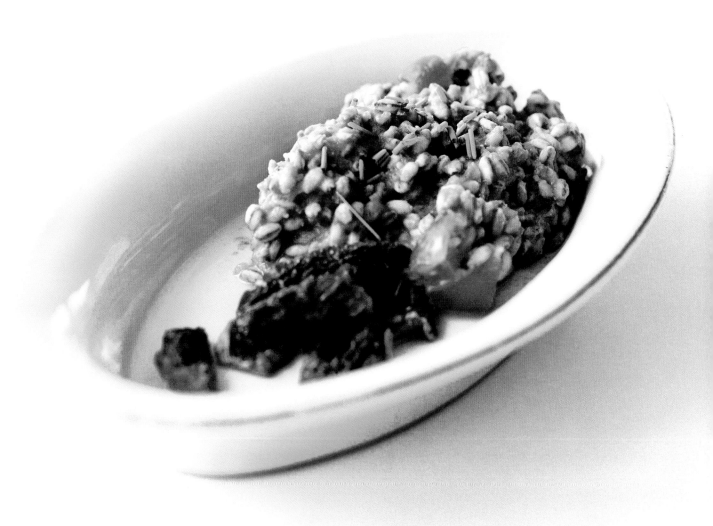

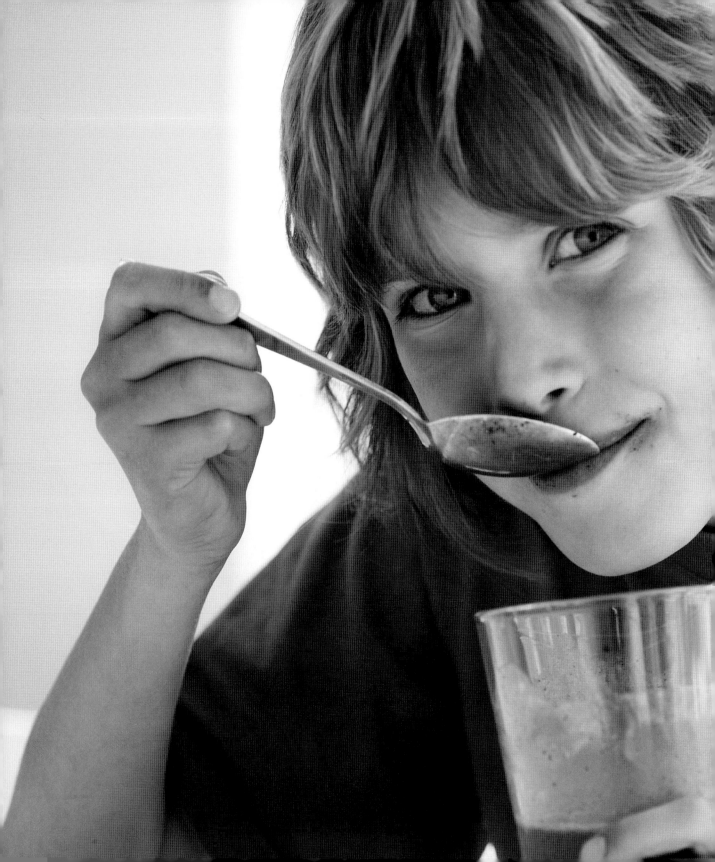

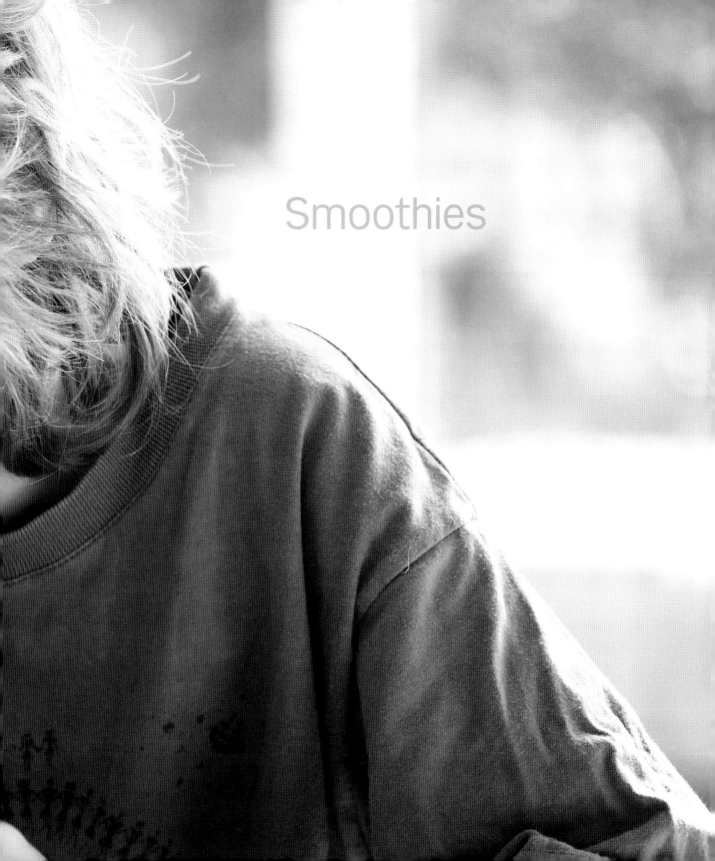

Smoothies

Some days I only live off smoothies. They taste heavenly and there are so many variations.

If you can't get ahold of raw cacao, use carob instead. Some people only use carob, but I don't like the taste. I prefer using ordinary good-quality, non-raw cacao powder such as Valrhona instead.

Some people like protein powder or oil in their smoothies. Personally, I'm not so keen on that, but it is a matter of taste. I prefer to use oil in dressings or as a shot with freshly squeezed juice.

Serve your smoothie in a large glass with a straw or try it in a wine glass or a cocktail glass. It looks more delicate served in a glass with a stem.

When you have ripe bananas, peel and slice them in about 1.5 inch (3 cm) long pieces, then freeze them. This way you always have bananas ready for delicious smoothies.

Vanilla or Cinnamon Smoothie

1¾ cups (4 dls) nut milk
Frozen bananas
2 teaspoons vanilla or cinnamon

Mix all in a blender until you have the most delicious, soft smoothie. The recipe doesn't say how much banana to use because people's tastes vary, and it is much easier for you to decide on your ideal portions. So make your smoothie as creamy or as light as you like it.

This is a basic smoothie recipe and it tastes delicious, especially if you fancy vanilla or cinnamon.

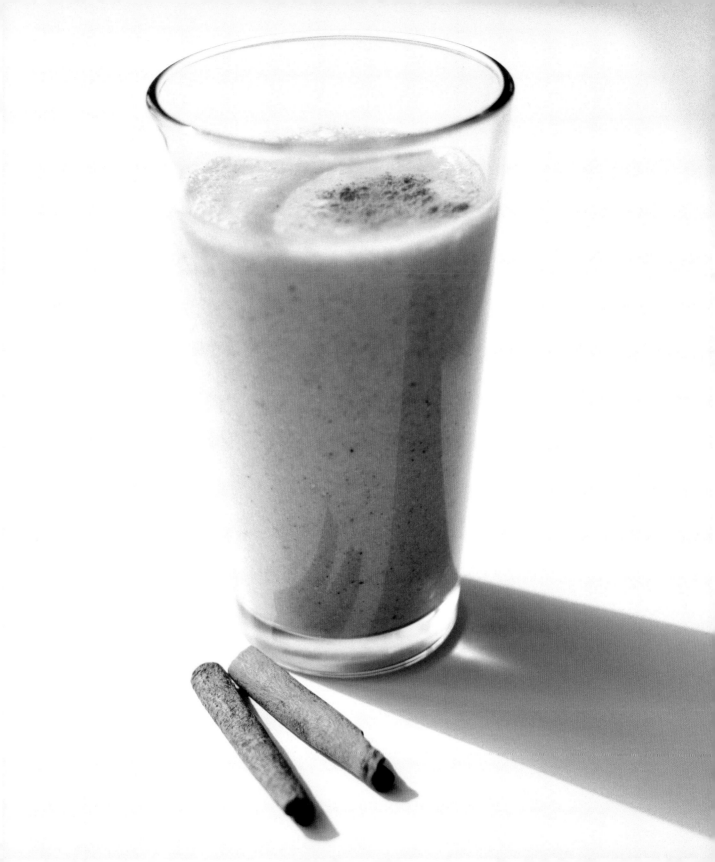

Orange-Raspberry Shake

2 oranges
1 banana
¾ cup (2 dls) raspberries
Agave nectar

Mix everything in a blender until you have the most delicious, soft smoothie.

You decide whether the banana or the raspberries should be frozen.

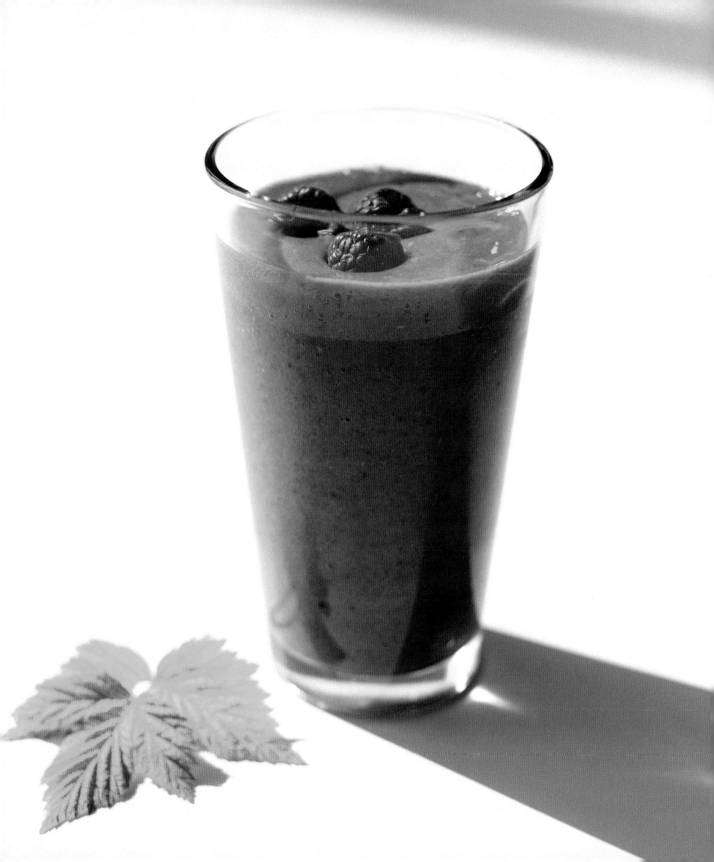

Yummy Blueberry-Strawberry Shake

1¼–1¾ cups (3–4 dls) nut milk
1 tablespoon honey
1 handful frozen strawberries
¾ cup (1½ dls) frozen blueberries
2 small ripe bananas or 1 large banana
½ tablespoon raw cacao
½ teaspoon vanilla or cardamom
1–2 tablespoons coconut oil

Mix all the ingredients in a blender until you have the most delicious, soft smoothie.

This recipe is a bit more complex, but the taste is enchanting and seductive.

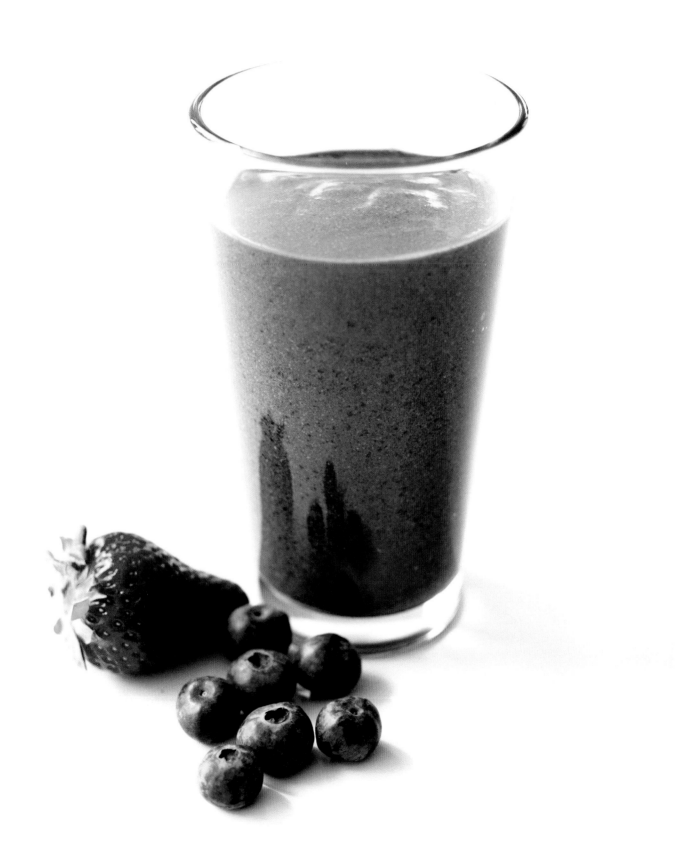

Chocolate Mint Shake

1 ripe avocado
1¼ cup (3 dls) nut milk
2–3 tablespoons cacao
2 tablespoons agave nectar
1 handful fresh mint leaves

Mix all ingredients in a blender until you have the most delicious, soft smoothie.

You can replace the avocado with a banana if you don't feel like using avocado in the smoothie.

One avocado is fantastic at getting that rich, creamy consistency, but don't use too much. You should not be able to taste the avocado.

Easy Chocolate Shake

½ guadeloupe melon
2 tablespoons agave nectar
1 tablespoon raw cacao powder

Remove seeds from the melon. Mix it with the other ingredients in a blender.

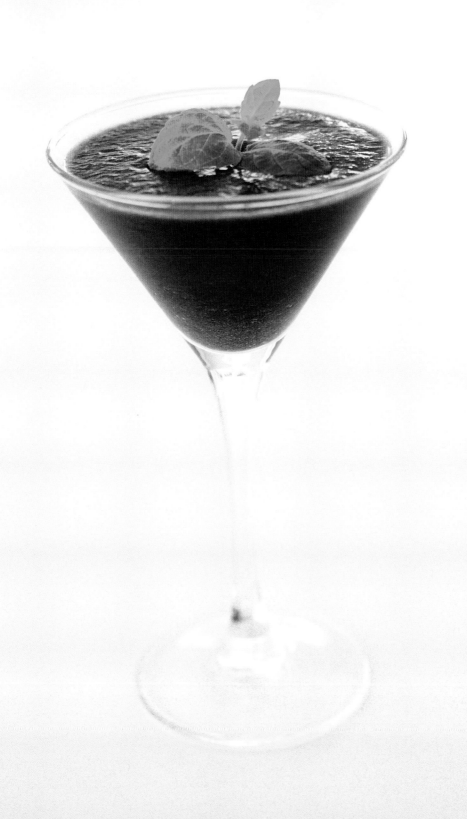

Orange and Black-currant Shake

2 oranges, peeled
¾ cup (2 dls) black currants, fresh or frozen
3–5 dates, pitted

Blend the dates, oranges, and black currants in a blender. You can add honey or more dates to the shake if it tastes too sour.

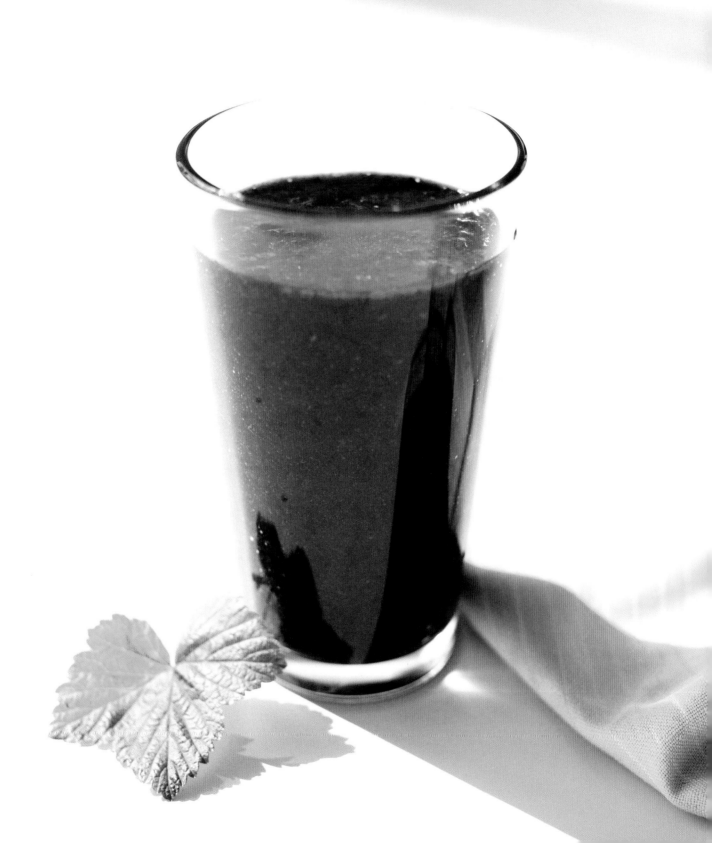

Blue Passion

1¾ cup (4 dls) pineapple
1¼ cup (3 dls) nut milk
2 tablespoons agave nectar
½ teaspoon vanilla

¾ cup (2 dls) blueberries
1 passion fruit

Blend the pineapple, nut milk, agave nectar, and vanilla. Pour the mixture into a champagne glass (or two) until it is half full.

Add the blueberries to the remaining mixture and blend, then add to the mixture in the half-filled glass.

Cut the passion fruit in half and remove the flesh with a spoon. Add the passion fruit and serve.

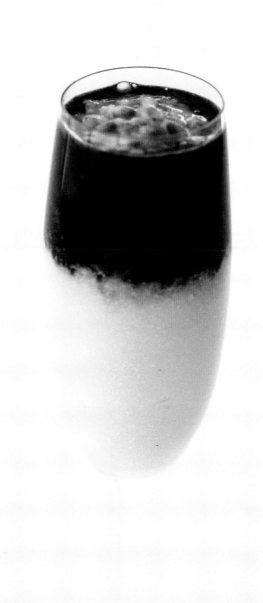

Strawberry-Banana Smoothie

If you have fresh strawberries, use frozen bananas, or else use frozen strawberries and ripe bananas.

1¾ cup (4 dls) nut milk
1–2 ripe bananas
1¾ cup (4 dls) frozen strawberries
1 teaspoon vanilla

Mix all the ingredients in a blender until deliciously smooth.

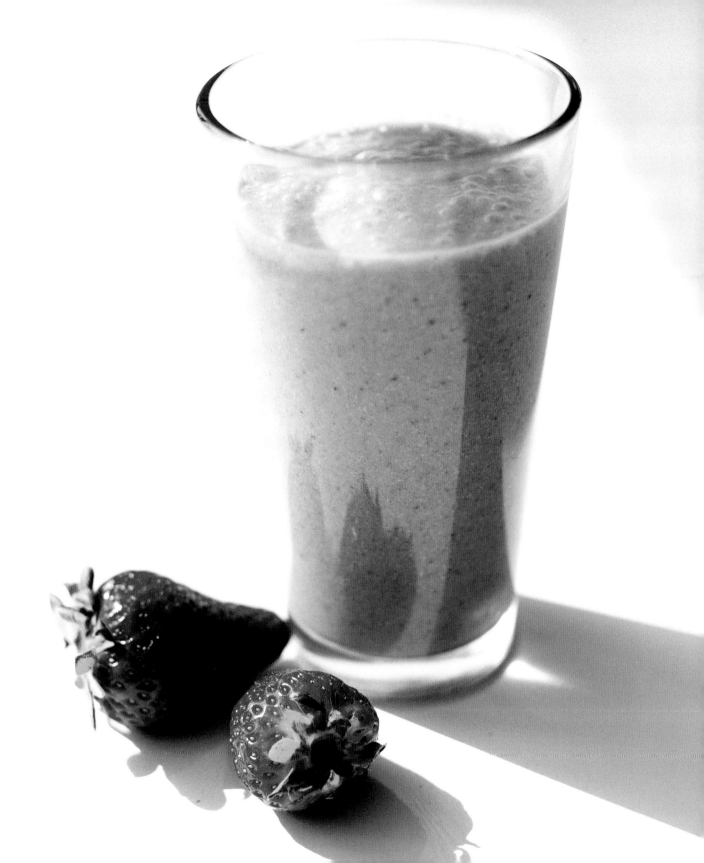

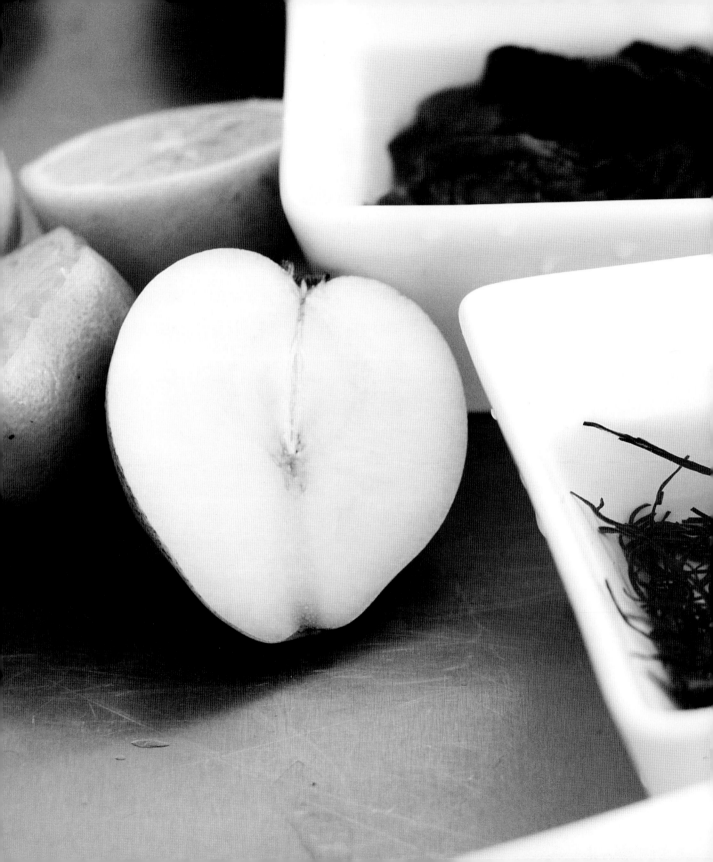

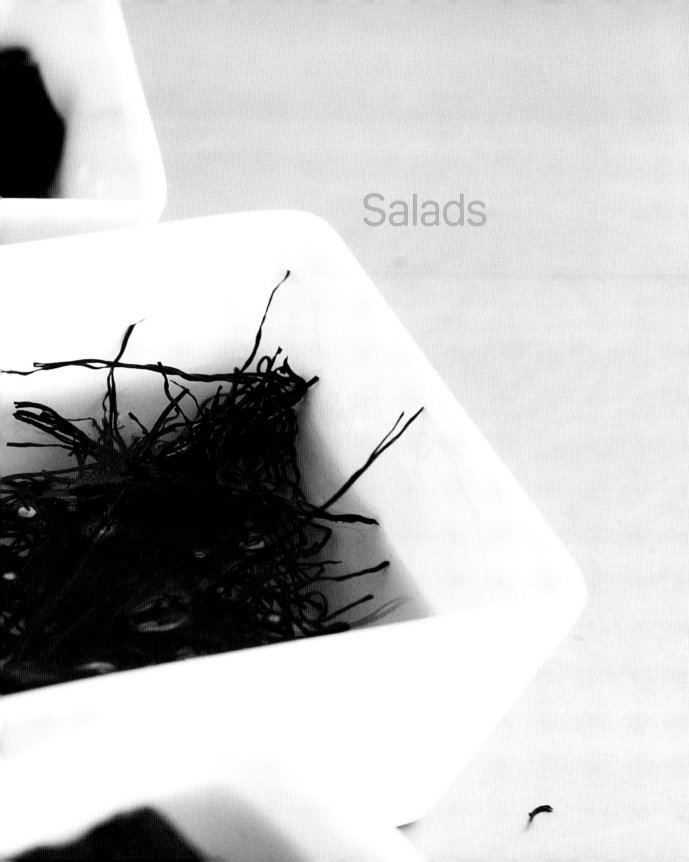

Salads

Beetroot in Horseradish Cream

3 large beetroots
2 apples

¾ cup (200 g) cashews
¾ cup (2 dls) water
2 tablespoons olive oil
2 tablespoons agave nectar
1 tablespoon onion

1–1.5 ounces (30–50g) grated horseradish
Salt and pepper

Capers (optional)

Peel and dice the beetroots and apples. Blend the other ingredients using a hand blender. Add salt, pepper, and more horseradish to taste.

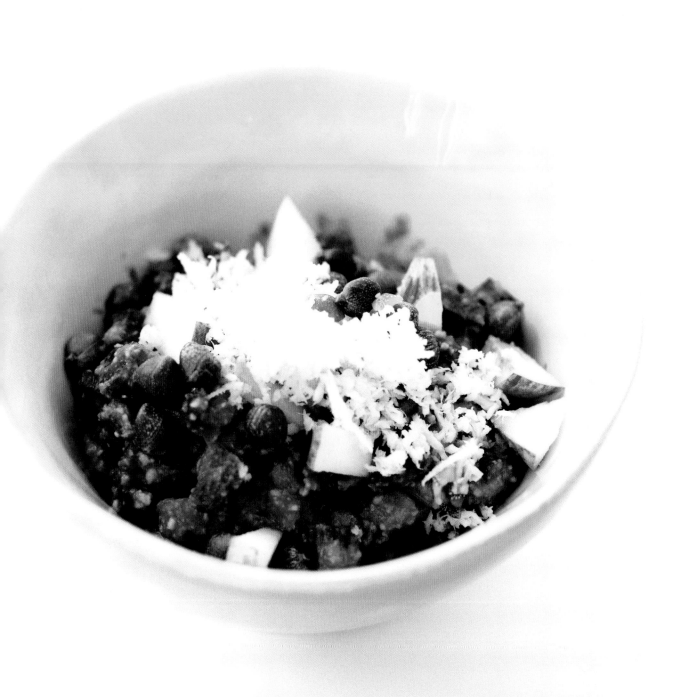

Seaweed Salad

2 tablespoons (30 g) arame seaweed

2 tablespoons (30 g) wakame seaweed

2 tablespoons (30 g) nori seaweed

1 cucumber

1 large beetroot

1 bunch of radishes

1 scallion

½ cup (¾ dl) sesame oil

Juice of ½ lemon

3 tablespoons agave nectar

2 tablespoons ginger

1 tablespoon Bragg Liquid Aminos or Nama Shoyu

3 tablespoons sesame seeds

Soak the seaweed until it is soft but still springy. To achieve the right "bite" in the different kinds of seaweed it is important that they soak separately. Drain seaweed and mix together in a bowl. Peel and julienne cucumber. Peel and grate the beetroot. Slice the radishes and julienne the scallion. Mix ingredients together carefully.

Blend the oil, lemon juice, nectar, ginger, and soy sauce using a hand blender.

Serve the salad on a plate, pour the dressing over it, and garnish with sesame seeds. This salad is best the day it is made.

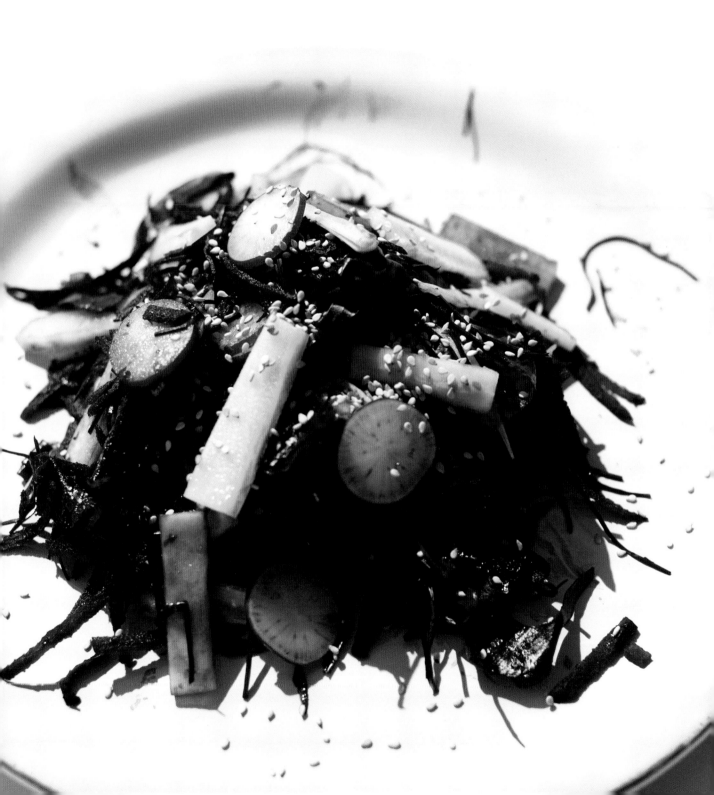

Fresh Asparagus

1 bunch of asparagus
Olive oil
Coarse salt

Hold each stalk of asparagus in your hands and bend it until it breaks. Only use the upper part. Arrange the stalks on a small plate, drizzle them with oil, and sprinkle with salt.

Can be served with olive tapenade (p. 192) or hummus (p. 188).

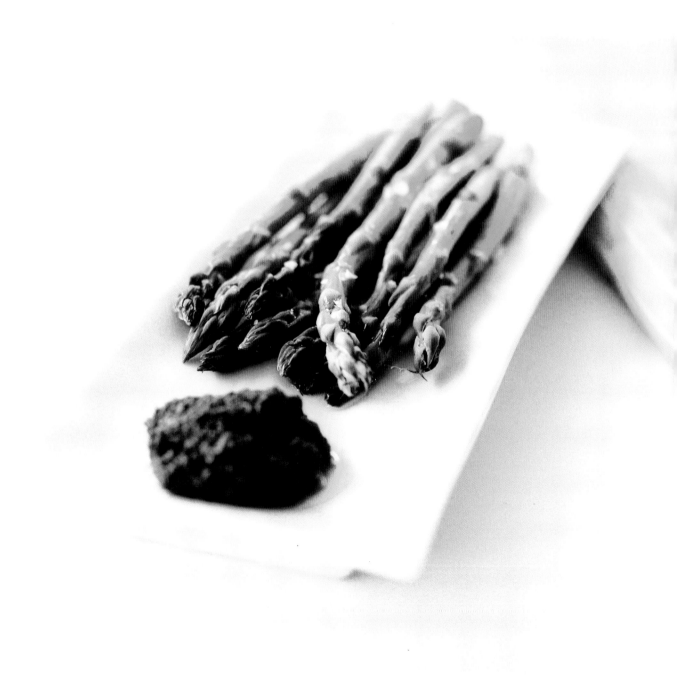

Basic Instinct

2 avocados
1 yellow bell pepper
½ cucumber
8 cherry tomatoes
¾ cup (2 dls) alfalfa sprouts
10.5 ounces (100 g) baby spinach
10 olives
6 sun-dried tomatoes, sliced
⅓ cup (¾ dl) pumpkin seeds

Dice avocados, bell pepper, and cucumber. Cut the tomatoes in half and combine with the other ingredients in a bowl.

Serve with olive oil and herbal salt or your favorite dressing.

See how easily you can dice an avocado on p. 289.

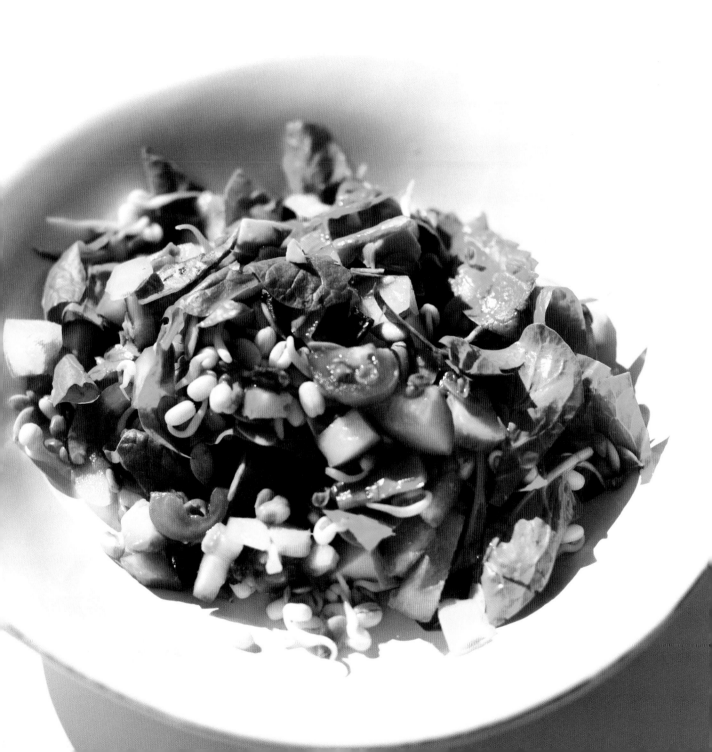

Cabbage Curry Salad

½ small green cabbage, finely chopped
½ apple, finely chopped

Curry Cream:
3½ tablespoons (50 g) cashews
1 tablespoon curry
1 teaspoon lemon juice
1 tablespoon apple cider vinegar
1 tablespoon water
Salt and pepper

Mix the cabbage and apple together in a bowl.

Using a hand blender, grind the nuts into flour. Add the curry, lemon juice, apple cider vinegar, and water. Blend again until you have a thick, fluid cream. Add salt and pepper to taste.

Carefully fold the curry cream into the cabbage-and-apple mixture.

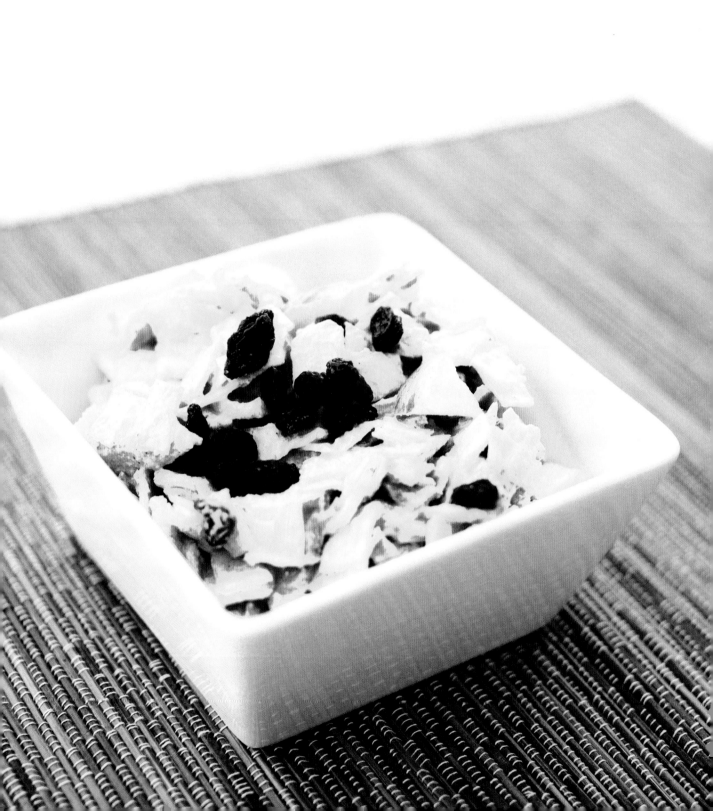

Orange and Red Cabbage Salad

½ small red cabbage, finely chopped
1 large orange, diced
3½ tablespoons (50 g) coarsely chopped hazelnuts

½ cup (1 dl) nutty oil or neutral-tasting oil
½ tablespoon Dijon mustard
1 tablespoon raw honey
2 tablespoons apple cider vinegar

In a bowl, combine the cabbage, orange pieces, and nuts.

Combine the other ingredients to make the dressing, stirring until smooth.

Toss the cabbage, orange, and nut mixture with the dressing.

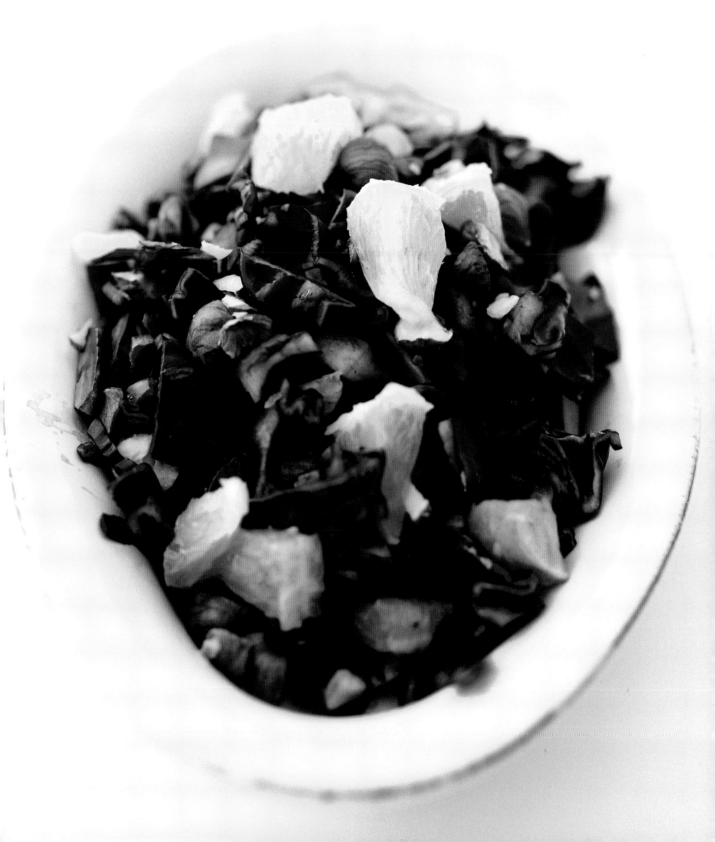

Bold Salad of Fennel, Red Grapefruit, and Avocado

2 red grapefruit
2 avocados
1 large fennel
½ cup (1 dl) mint leaves
1 tablespoon lime juice
½ cup (1 dl) nut oil or neutral-tasting oil
1 teaspoon crushed coriander
Salt and pepper

Cut the grapefruit into segments. Cut the avocado into slices and julienne the fennel. Mix all the ingredients in a bowl (leaving a few mint leaves for garnishing) and serve on a plate.

This salad is both attractive and delicious!

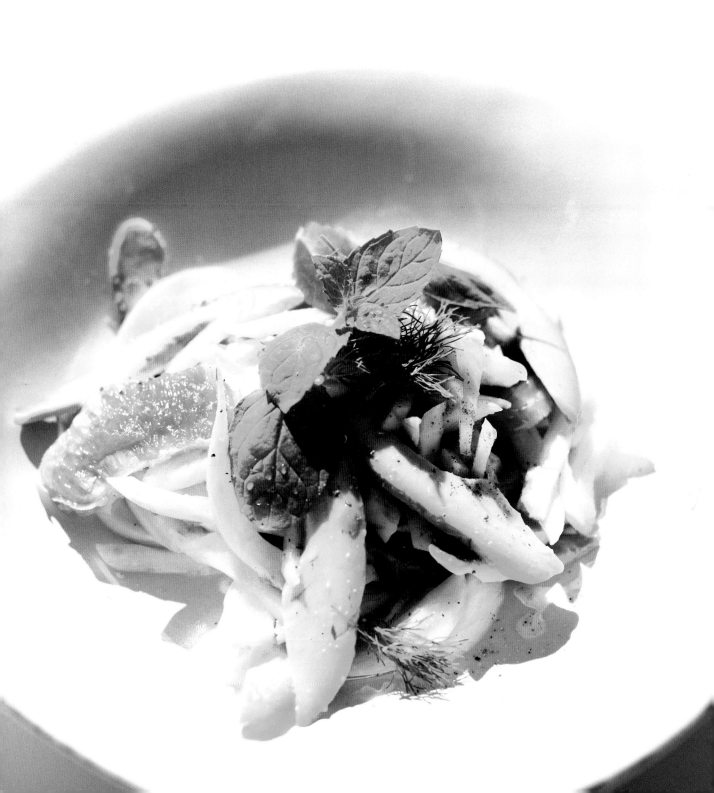

Arugula Salad with Pears

½ cup (125 g) arugula or baby spinach
1 large pear
Juice of 1 lime
⅓ cup (¾ dl) neutral-tasting oil
2 tablespoons raw honey

½ cup (1 dl) sun-dried goji berries
½ cup (1 dl) pumpkin seeds
Salt and pepper

Rinse the greens and remove stems. Peel the pear and remove the core. Use a potato peeler to cut the pear into paper-thin slices.

Mix the lime juice, oil, and honey with a hand blender. Toss the salad and pear with the dressing.

Serve on a plate and garnish with goji berries and pumpkin seeds. Add freshly ground pepper and coarse salt to taste.

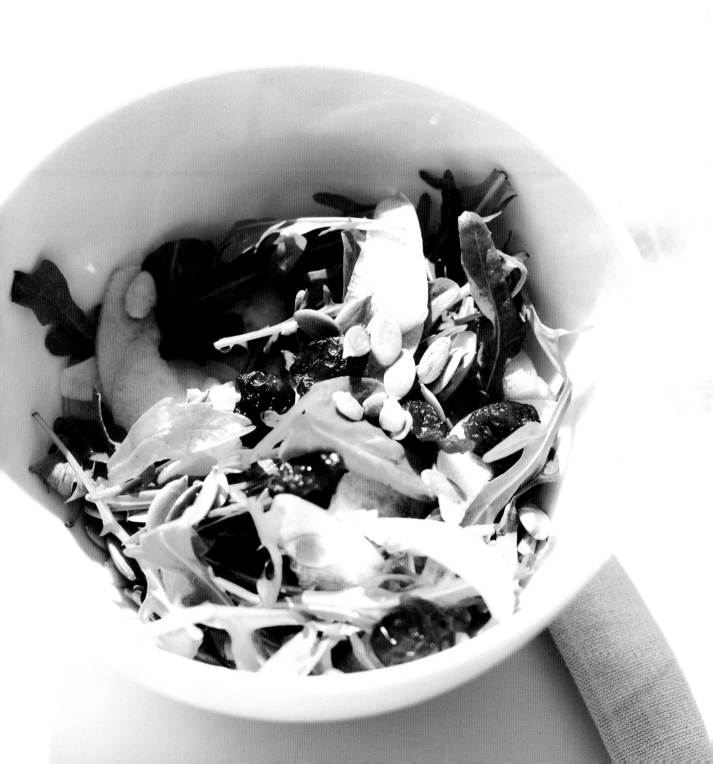

Root Vegetable Salad

2 cups (500 g) parsnips
1¼ cups (300 g) Jerusalem artichoke
8 sun-dried tomatoes, sliced
1 handful chopped parsley

¼ red onion
¾ cup (1½ dls) olive oil
4 teaspoons Dijon mustard
3 teaspoons raw honey
Salt and pepper

Peel and dice the parsnips and artichoke and mix them together in a large bowl with the sun-dried tomatoes and most of the chopped parsley (save some for garnish).

Blend the onion, oil, mustard, and honey using a hand blender. Add salt and pepper to taste. Toss the dressing and root vegetables together and place the salad in the refrigerator to marinate for a few hours.

Serve garnished with parsley.

You can use all kinds of root vegetables. Instead of chopping the parsley with a knife, you can put it in a large glass and cut it with scissors.

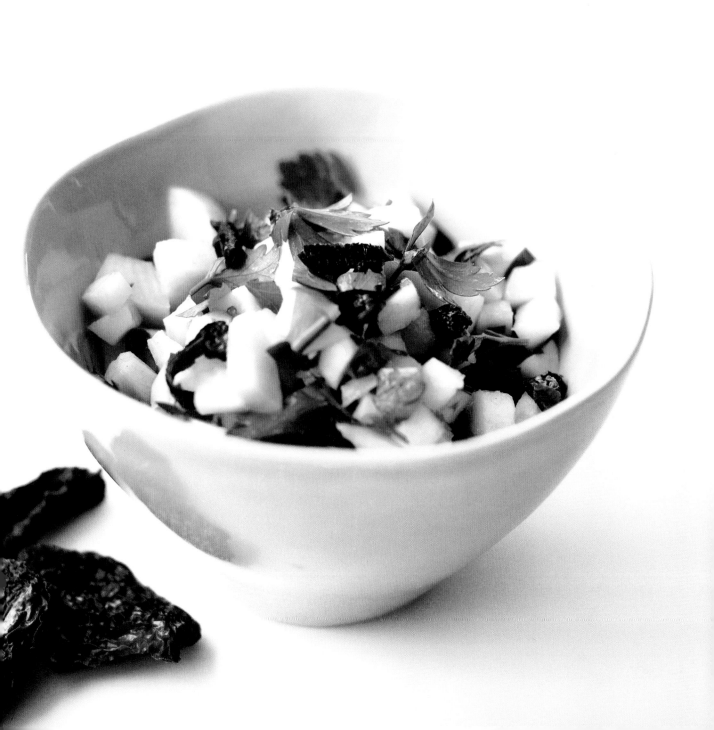

Waldorf Salad

3 stalks celery
2 apples
⅓ cup (75 g) walnuts, coarsely chopped

⅔ cup (150 g) cashews
½ cucumber, diced
2 tablespoons neutral-tasting oil
1 teaspoon apple cider vinegar
Salt

10 black grapes, halved

Dice the celery and apples and mix with the walnuts. Blend the cashews, cucumber, oil, vineger, and salt to taste with a hand blender.

Garnish with the grapes.

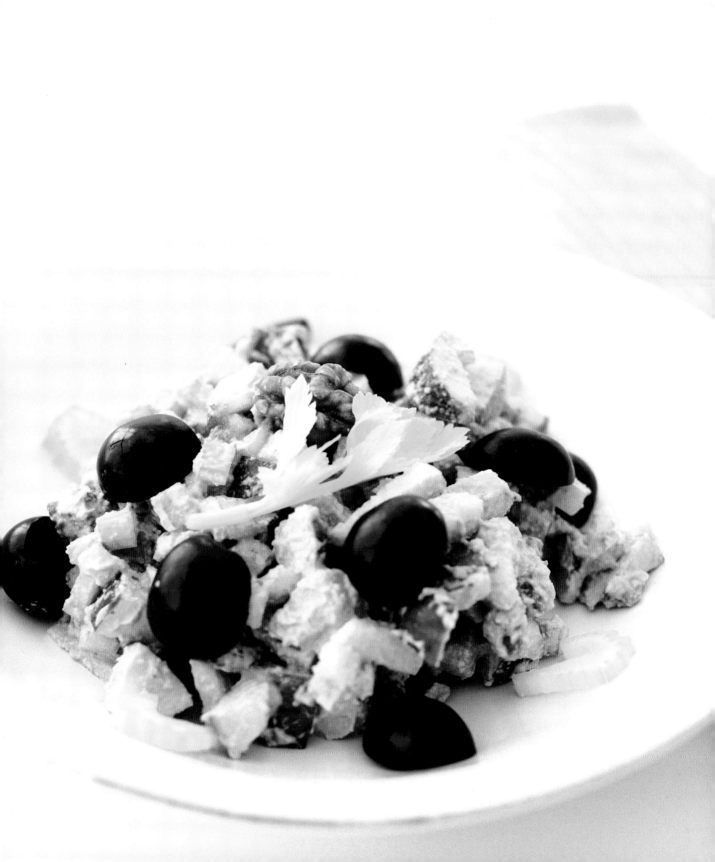

Salad with Walnuts and Fennel

1 handful radicchio
1 handful lamb's lettuce (mâche), or other lettuce
½ fennel bulb
Juice of ½ orange
2 tablespoons (30 g) walnuts

Tear radicchio and lettuce into small pieces. Julienne the fennel and mix with the greens.

Pour the orange juice over the salad and garnish with walnuts.

Try soaking the julienned fennel in orange juice for a few hours before mixing it into the salad. You will probably need a little more orange juice for soaking.

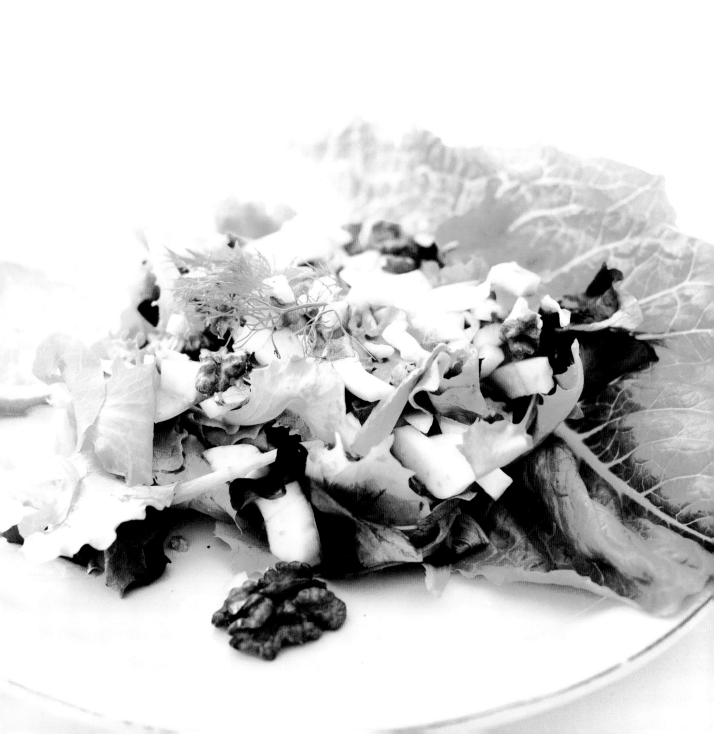

Broccoli and Kale on a Bed of Red Cabbage

Marinade:
2 handfuls kale, destemmed
¾ cup (1½ dl) mix of sesame oil and rapeseed oil
½ cup (1 dl) water
3 tablespoons lemon or lime juice
2 garlic cloves
2 teaspoons Bragg Liquid Aminos, Nama Shoyu, or ½ teaspoon salt
Cayenne

1 ear of corn or 3.5 ounces (100 g) frozen corn
½ head of broccoli florets
1 handful chopped red cabbage
1 small red onion, chopped

Red cabbage leaves
2 tablespoons chopped hazelnuts

Mix all the ingredients for the marinade and blend until creamy and green. Add cayenne to taste.

Cut corn kernels off the cob and put them in a bowl with the broccoli florets, red cabbage, and chopped onion, and toss with the marinade. Let it rest for at least 2 hours. Use a colander to strain off the marinade and save it.

Place the cabbage leaves on a plate and arrange the vegetables on top. Garnish with nuts and serve the marinade as extra dressing.

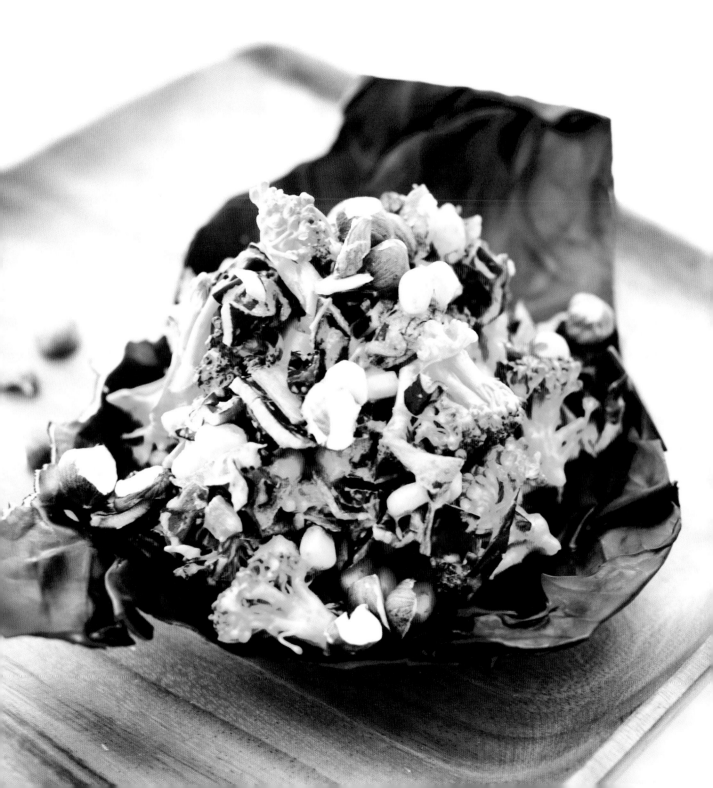

Tomato and Avocado Salad

4 tomatoes
2 ripe avocados
12 black olives
Salt and pepper
Olive oil
Fresh basil

Cut the tomato and avocado into slices and arrange on a small plate, alternating tomato with avocado. Cut the olives in half, remove the pits, and arrange the olives around the tomato and avocado. Garnish with coarse salt and freshly ground pepper. Carefully pour olive oil over the dish and garnish with lots of basil leaves.

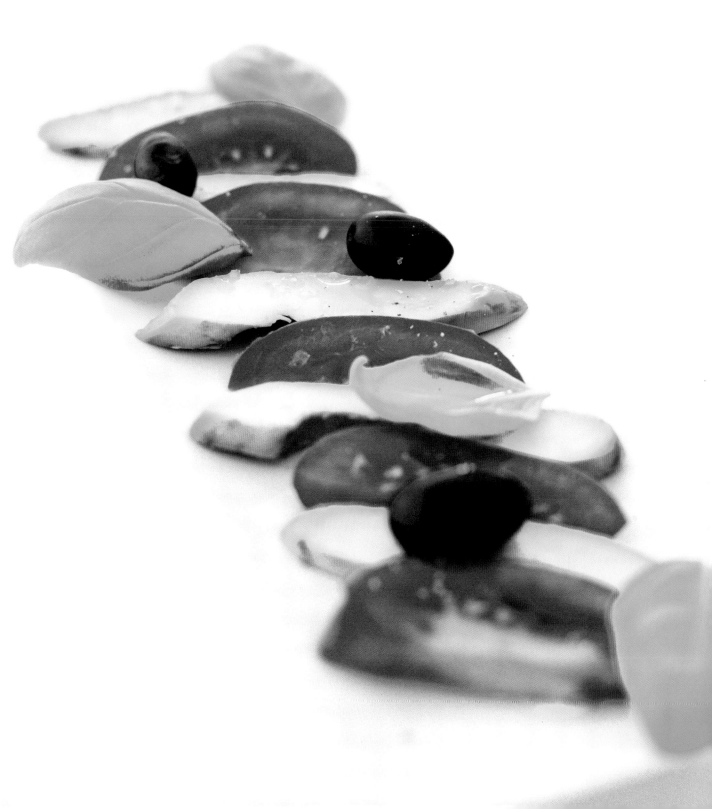

Greek Salad with Tzatziki

¾ head romaine lettuce

10 radishes

½ cucumber

2 tomatoes, coarsely chopped

1 small red onion, finely chopped

10 kalamata olives, pitted

1 small handful parsley, finely chopped

1 small handful mint, finely chopped

3½ tablespoons (50 g) cashews

Tzatziki (p. 184)

Tear the lettuce into small pieces and cut the radishes and cucumber into slices. Combine all the ingredients and garnish with cashews.

Serve on a plate with tzatziki on the side or mixed with tzatziki.

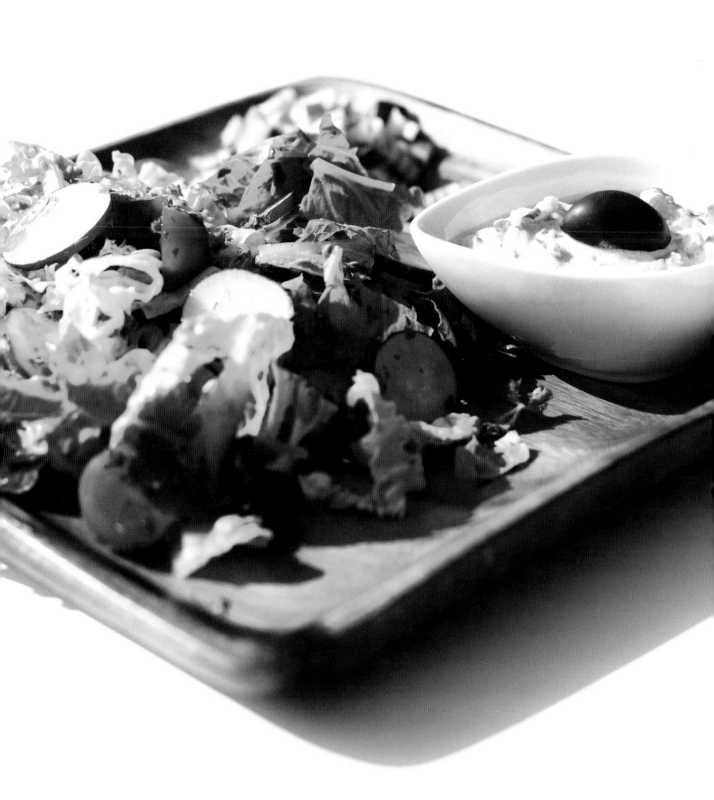

Papaya Salad

¼ head iceberg lettuce
½ papaya
1 red bell pepper
2 avocados
2 carrots

4 tablespoons Udo's Choice Oil Blend
½ lime
¼ teaspoon cumin

1¼ cup (1½ dls) arame seaweed
3 tablespoons sunflower seeds

Cut the lettuce, papaya, red bell pepper, and avocado into strips. Use a peeler to make the carrot strips. Make the dressing with oil, lime juice, and cumin.

Arrange the strips of lettuce, papaya, red bell pepper, avocados, and carrots with the seaweed on a plate, pour the dressing on top, and garnish with sunflower seeds.

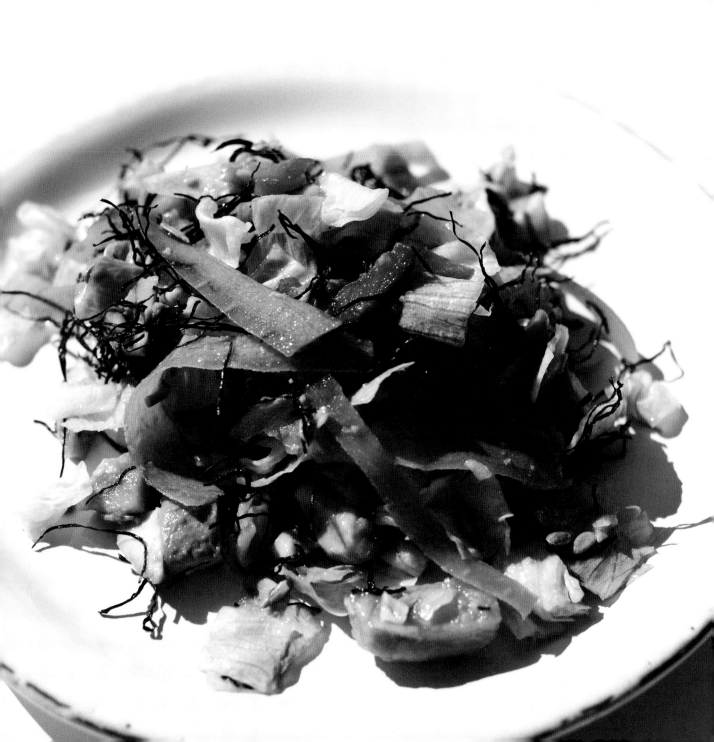

Egg Salad Look-alike

3 avocados
3 sun-dried tomatoes

Curry cream (p. 90)

Dice the avocado and chop the sun-dried tomatoes. Gently fold in the curry cream until well combined, taking care not to crush the avocado.

See how easily you can dice an avocado on p. 289.

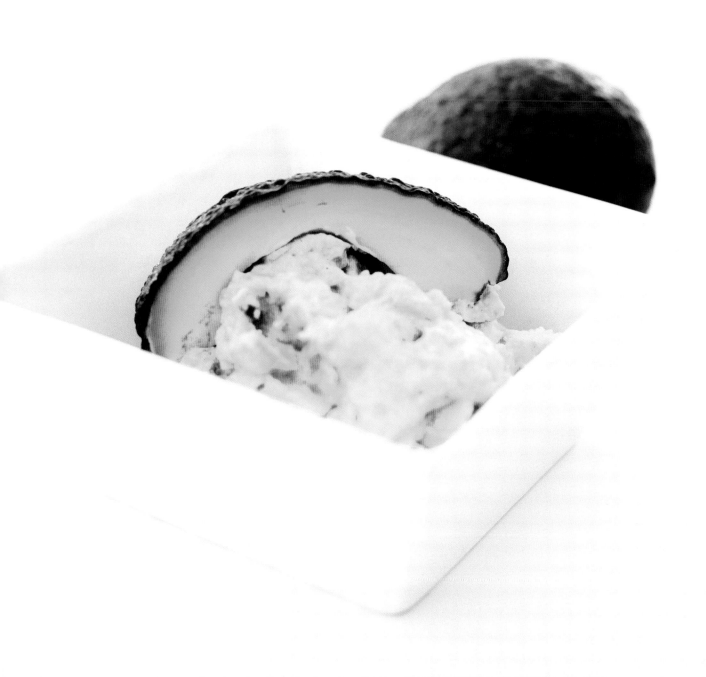

Stuffed Tomato Hors D'oeuvres

20 cherry tomatoes
4–5 different dips or pâtés (e.g., leftovers)

Cut off the tops of the tomatoes and remove the "meat" with a teaspoon. Fill the tomatoes with dips or pâté (p. 180).

Serve on a dish as a first course or as pure self-indulgence.

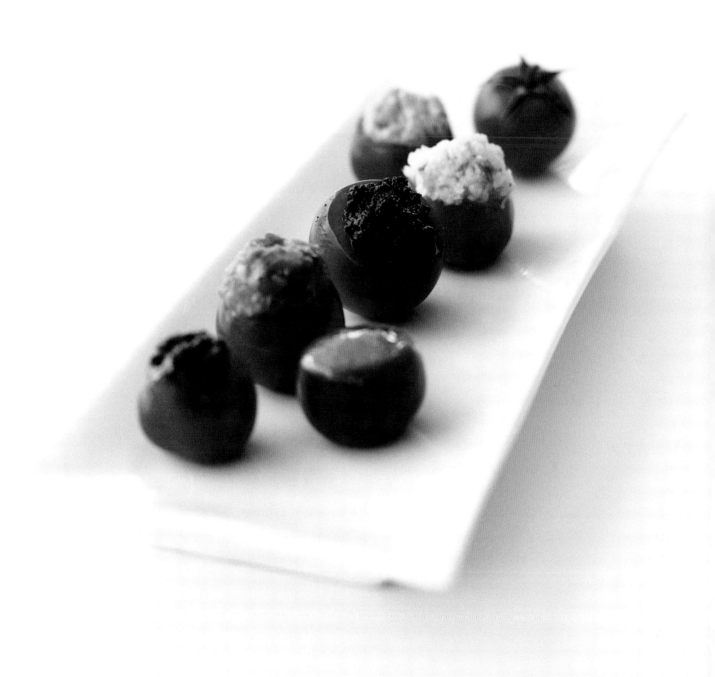

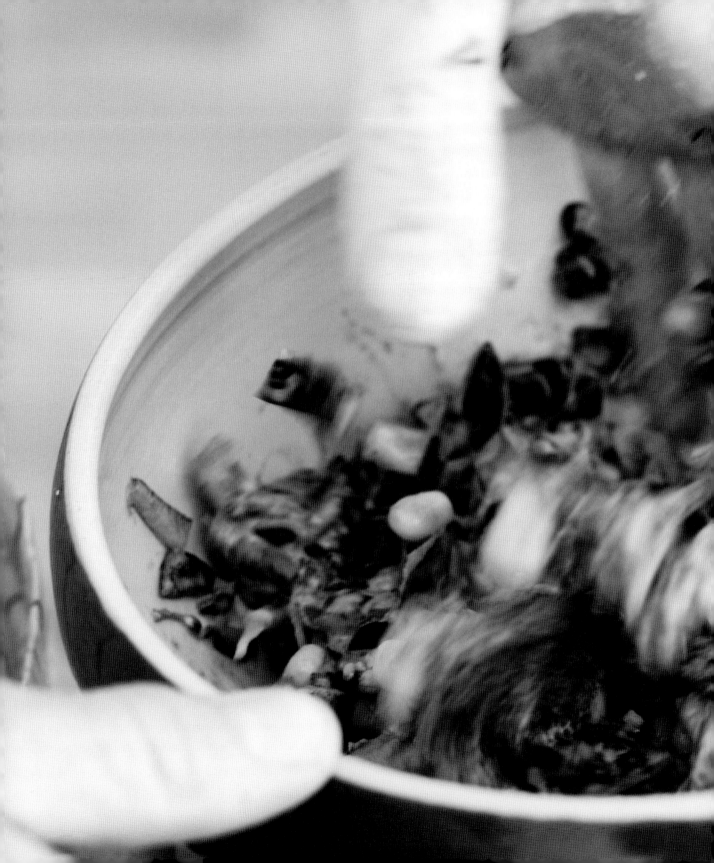

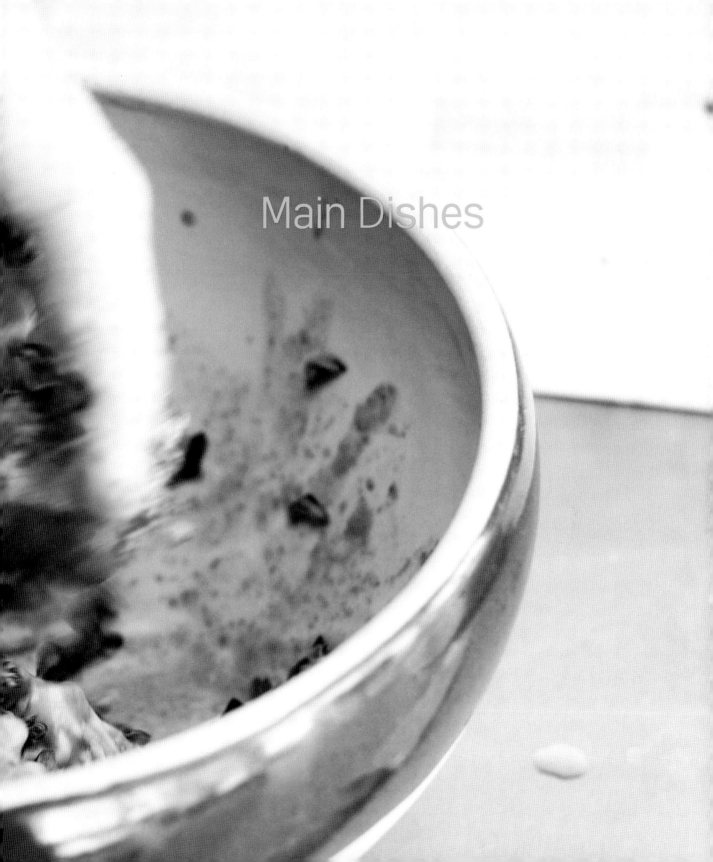

Main Dishes

Not Stir-fried

1 squash
1 carrot
1 red pepper
½–1 cup (1–2 dls) chopped broccoli florets
1 handful finely chopped white cabbage or red cabbage
2 tablespoons sesame oil
1 tablespoon Bragg Liquid Aminos or Nama Shoyu

Asian sweet chili sauce (p. 279)

Sesame seeds

Finely grate the squash either with a spiral slicer or with a grater. Julienne the carrot and red pepper. Mix all the ingredients together in a bowl.

You will achieve the best results by leaving the mixture for an hour, occasionally stirring carefully so that the soy sauce and oil can marinate all the vegetables.

Serve on a plate with Asian sweet chili sauce and garnish with sesame seeds.

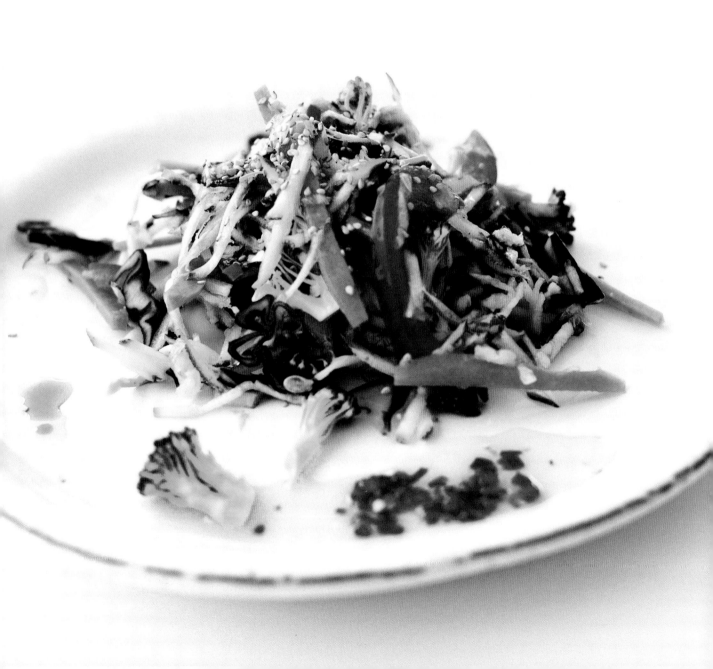

Lasagna

1 eggplant or 3 squash
½ cup (1 dl) olive oil
4 beefsteak tomatoes
½ cup (100 g) spinach

Béchamel sauce (p. 279)
Basic tomato sauce (p. 280)

1 handful fresh basil

Cut the eggplant into thin lasagna sheets. Marinate the eggplant slices in oil for 10 minutes. Cut the tomatoes into slices and coarse-chop the spinach. Arrange the eggplant slices on a plate and top with alternating layers of tomatoes, spinach, béchamel sauce, and tomato sauce. You can use the basil as garnish or put it into the lasagna.

You can vary the lasagna by using pesto instead of either the tomato sauce or béchamel sauce.

You can also blend the mixture with walnut meatloaf (p. 144) if you want the lasagna to be heavier.

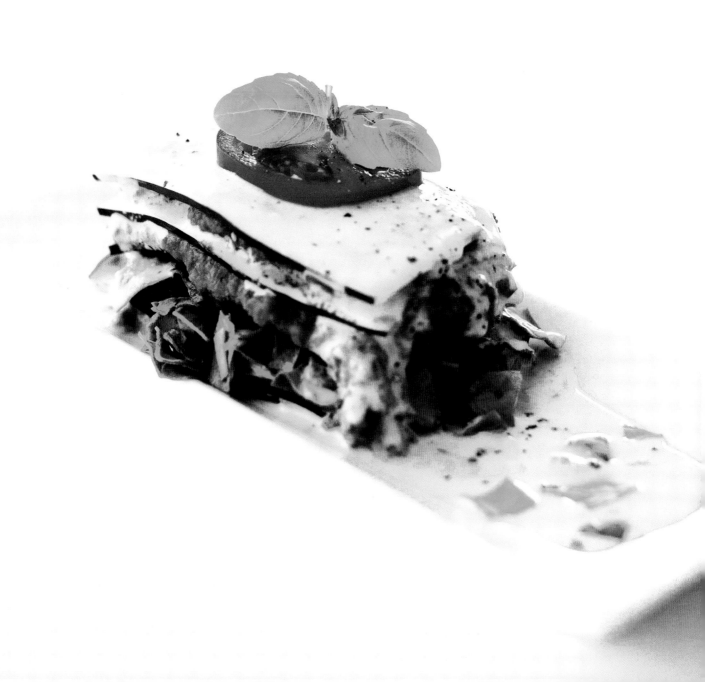

Sushi

½ head of cauliflower
4 nori sheets
Red cabbage crunch (p. 202)
Pea pâté (p. 202)
2 teaspoons cashew butter or peanut butter
1 carrot, peeled and julienned
Wasabi

Bragg Liquid Aminos or Nama Shoyu

Blend the cauliflower in a food processor until the consistency is like sticky rice.

Place one nori sheet on your sushi mat and arrange the "rice" on the sheet, leaving about a ¾ inch (2 cm) strip of nori uncovered at the far end (to be used for closing the sushi roll).

Arrange a strip of red cabbage crunch across the nori sheet, about ⅓ of the way into the sheet and about ¾ inch (2 cm) long. Top with same amount of pea pâté.

Finally, spread nut butter on a couple of carrot pieces and place them with the nut butter downward on the pâté.

Roll the nori sheet tightly and moisten the end of the sheet with a little water. Now you should have a whole roll of nori. Repeat until you have four rolls.

Cut each roll into 8–10 pieces and garnish each piece with a bit of wasabi. Serve with soy sauce.

You can see the whole process on p. 288.

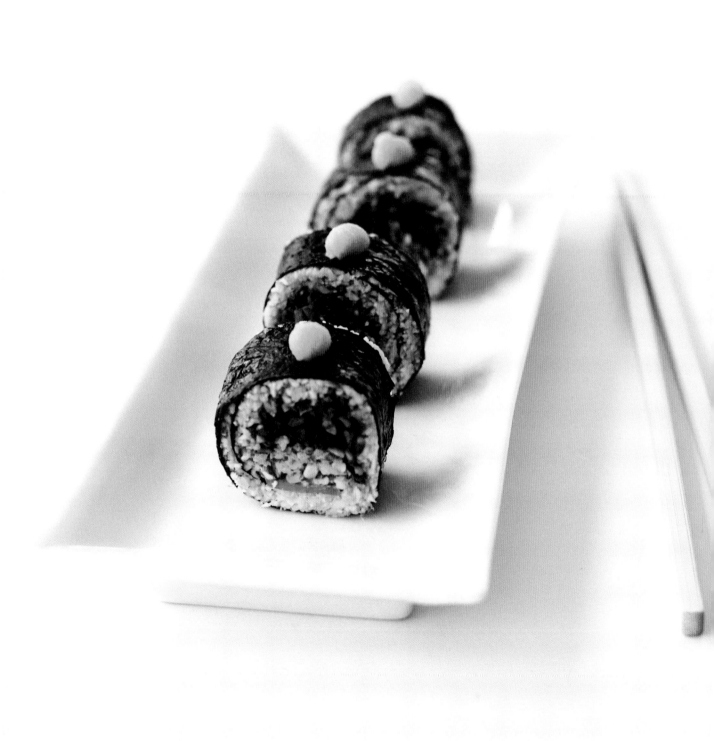

Pad Thai

1 squash
¼ cup (50 g) sugar peas
1 handful cashews
1 lime
1 handful bean sprouts
Pad Thai sauce (p. 278)

Grate the squash finely, either with a spiral slicer or with a grater. Slice the sugar peas finely, chop the cashews, and cut the lime into small wedges.

Arrange the squash and bean sprouts on a plate and top with sugar peas. Spoon the sauce over and garnish with nuts. Serve with a lime wedge, which can be squeezed onto the dish before eating.

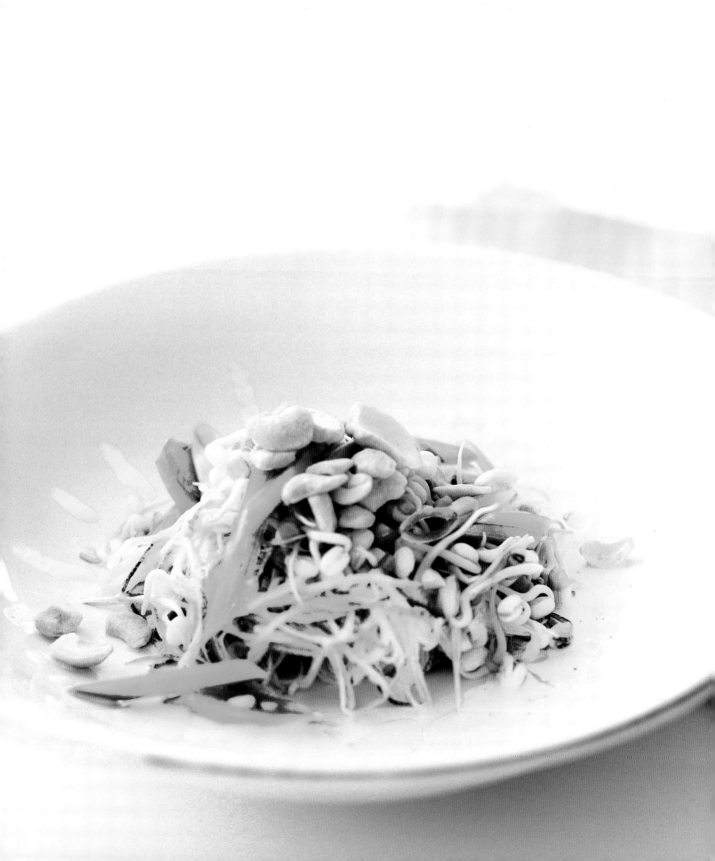

Thai Vegetables

Half a head of broccoli

¼ cabbage (red cabbage, savoy cabbage, or any other cabbage)

1 handful cashews

3 tablespoons Asian sweet chili sauce (p. 279)

Bragg Liquid Aminos or Nama Shoyu

½ cup pineapple, chopped (optional)

Finely chop the broccoli florets and cabbage. Mix all ingredients together and serve.

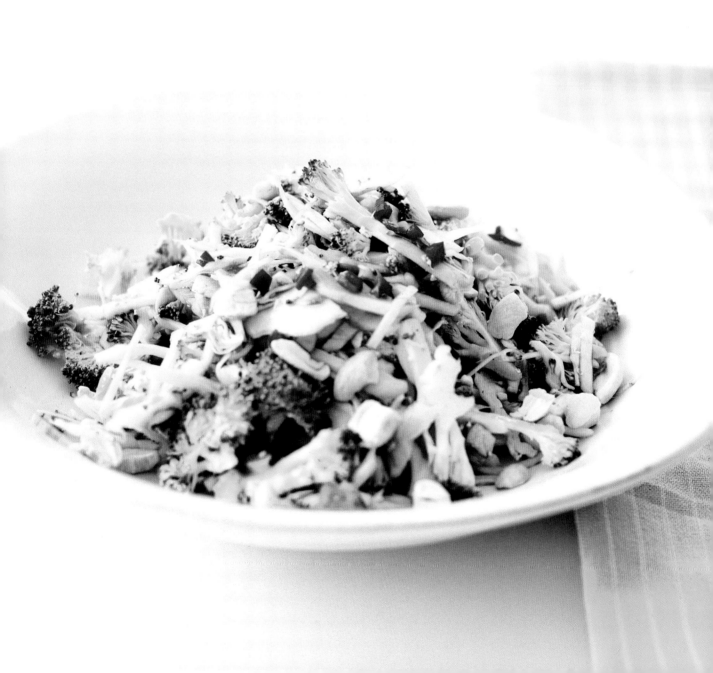

Spanish Rice

1¼ cups (300 g) wild rice, soaked 12 hours and
   sprouted 2 days (spelt can also be used)
2 chopped tomatoes
2 tablespoons chopped parsley
2 tablespoons olive oil
½ finely chopped red onion
1 teaspoon salt
3 teaspoons cumin

Cayenne
Lime

Wannabe Refried Beans

1¼ cups (3 dls) sunflower seeds
¾ cup (2 dls) sun-dried tomatoes
Juice of 1 lime
2 tablespoons olive oil
1 tablespoon agave nectar
2 teaspoons cumin
½–1 teaspoon cayenne pepper
1 teaspoon salt
(Extra water)

½ fresh chili pepper
2 scallions
2 teaspoons coriander

Garnish: Cilantro

Spanish Rice   Mix together the first seven ingredients and add cayenne and lime juice to taste. Marinate for a couple of hours to allow the flavors to blend.

Wannabe Refried Beans   Soak sunflower seeds for 2 hours and soak sun-dried tomatoes for 1 hour.

Mix all the ingredients except chili pepper, scallions, and coriander in a food processor. Blend until you have a thick and creamy mixture. Add a little water if the consistency is too thick.

Finely chop the chili pepper and scallion, add the coriander, and mix with the other ingredients.

Serving suggestion: Arrange on a dish with easy guacamole (p. 198) or place the mixture in hollowed peppers and serve with tomato sauce.

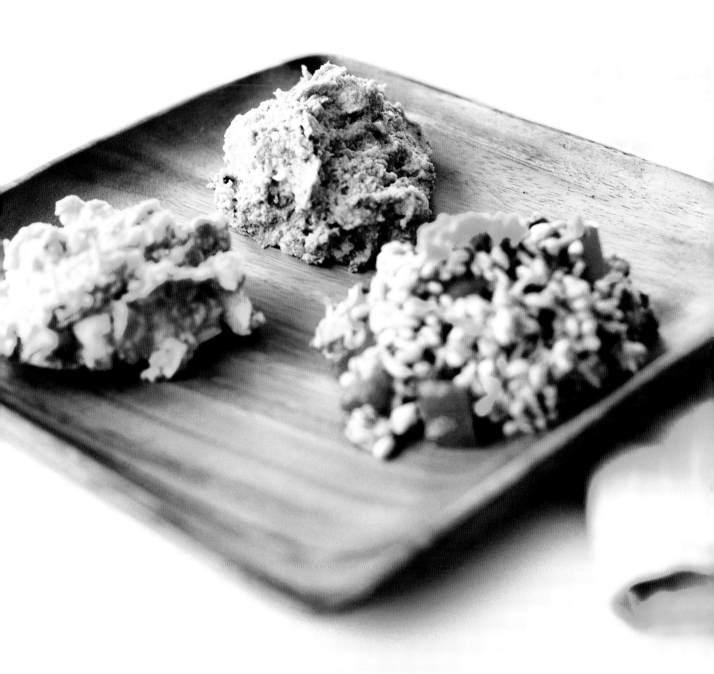

Sushi with "Salmon" Stuffing

Look-alike salmon pâté (p. 200)
4 nori sheets
Wasabi
Bragg Liquid Aminos, Nama Shoyu, or soy sauce
Thin slices of apple

Here is another of my favorites: sushi filled with look-alike salmon pâté. Prepare using the same procedure as the sushi on page 288. In this version, you replace the pea pâté and the red cabbage crunch with look-alike salmon pâté, and instead of carrots with nut butter, you top off with thin slices of apple.

There are many more ways of filling the nori sheets. Try using your favorite stuffing or simplify by using a variety of vegetables julienne as fillings.

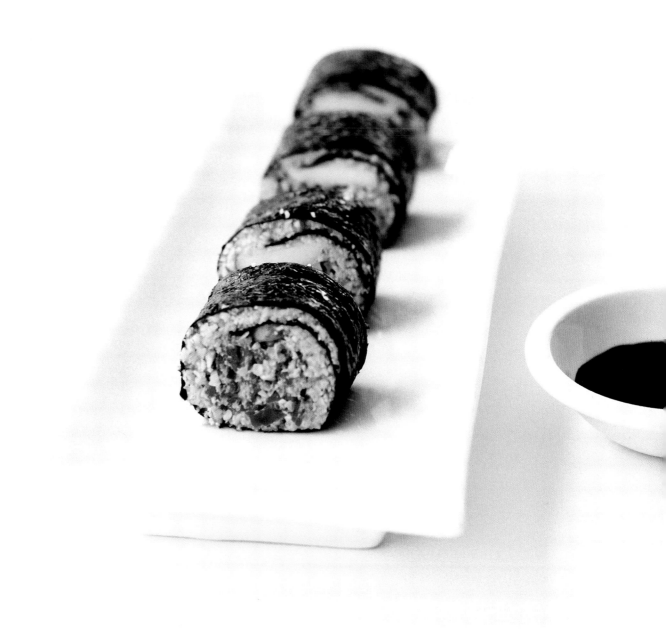

Lentils on Romaine Lettuce

¾ cup (180 g) lentils, soaked for 8 hours and sprouted 3 days
1 tomato, chopped
½ cucumber, chopped
½ yellow bell pepper, chopped
1 carrot, grated
Juice of ½ lemon
½ bunch of parsley, basil, or coriander

Cayenne
Crushed cumin
Salt and pepper
6 romaine lettuce leaves

Mix all the ingredients together in a bowl. Add cayenne, cumin, salt, and pepper to taste; maybe a drop of olive oil.

Arrange the lentil salad in portions on the lettuce leaves.

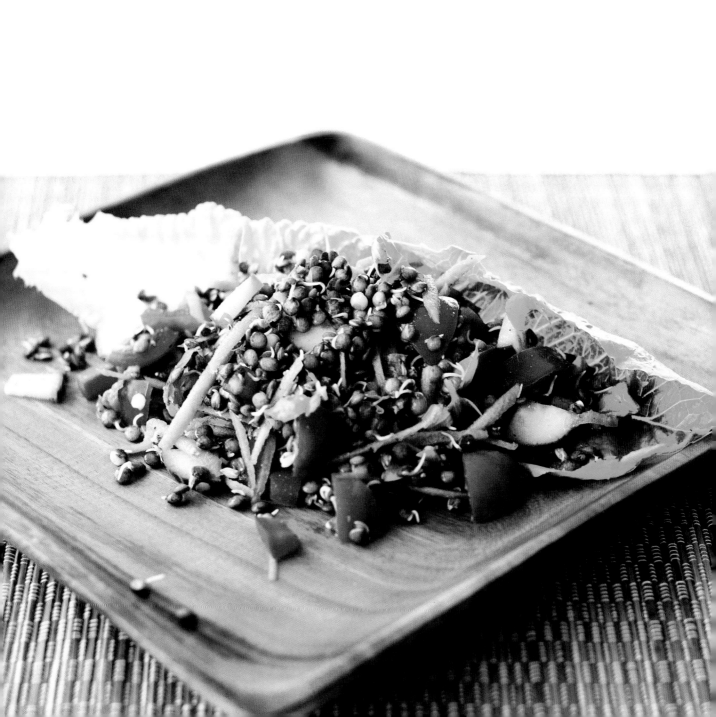

Cabbage Slaw

½ small white cabbage
1 carrot
1 handful parsley
½ cup (1 dl) raisins or cranberries
½ cup (1 dl) "You Just Might Think It's Crème Fraîche" (p. 262)
2 tablespoons tahini
Salt and pepper

Chop the cabbage finely. Grate the carrot and chop the parsley. Stir the sour cream and tahini together, adding the parsley, salt, and pepper. Mix all the ingredients, including the raisins, together in a bowl.

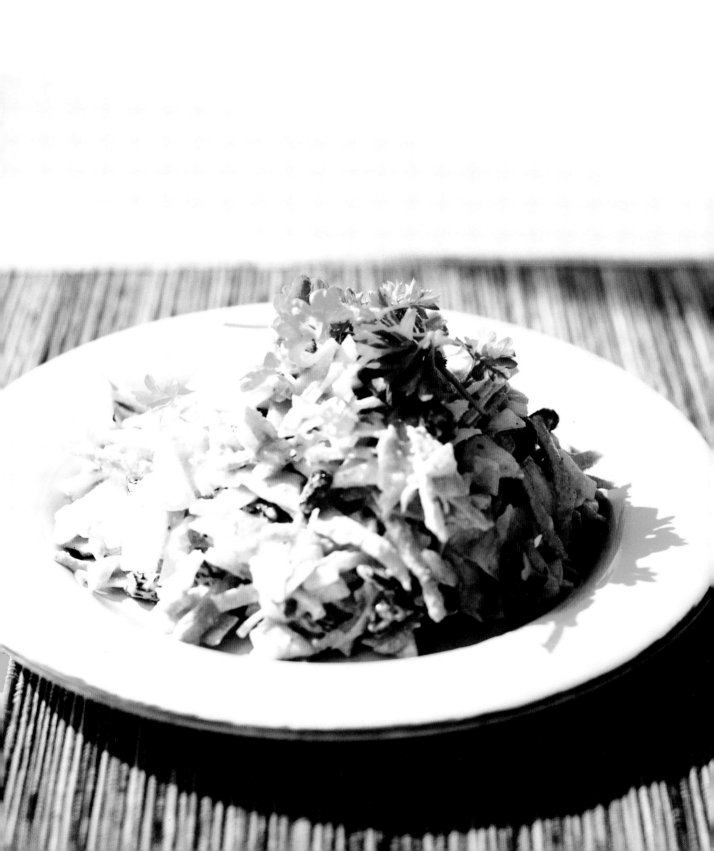

Middle Eastern Cauliflower Plate

This is very similar to the classic bulgur salad.

½ head of cauliflower
1 cucumber
1 red onion
½ cup (1 dl) cashews
¾ cup (150 g) dried apricots
1 cup (250 g) cherry tomatoes

½ cup (1 dl) olive oil
2 tablespoons lemon juice
1 handful chopped mint
1 handful chopped parsley
1 handful chopped coriander
Salt and pepper

Put the cauliflower in a food processor and blend until finely chopped. Finely chop the cucumber, onion, cashews, and apricots. Slice the tomatoes into halves. Mix all the ingredients together in a bowl.

Put the dressing ingredients into the blender and blend lightly. Add the dressing to the salad mixture and sprinkle herbs, salt, and pepper to taste.

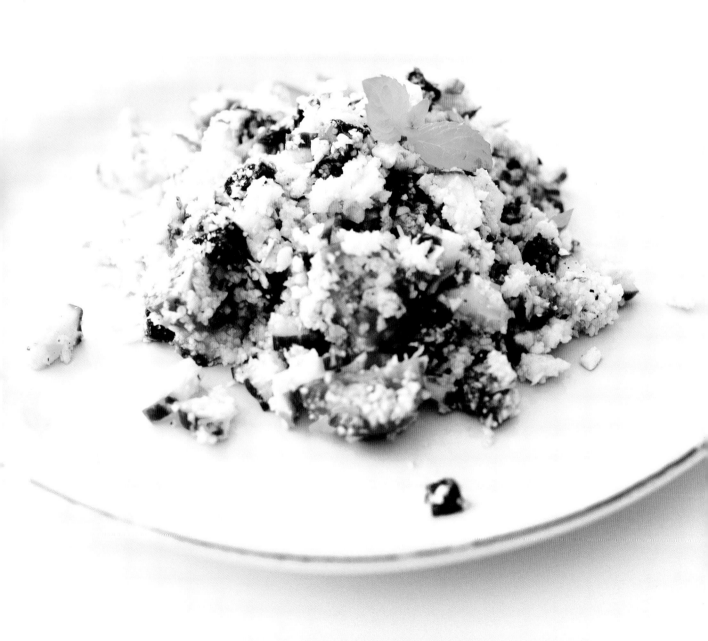

Pasta Pesto

1 large squash
1 small sweet potato
1 handful black olives
Pesto (pg. 196)
Fresh basil and finely chopped cashews (optional)

There are many ways of making pasta, and there are several vegetables that are suitable. Here I have chosen green squash in combination with a sweet potato. I prefer using a spiral slicer, which I bought abroad. If you don't have one, you can use an old-fashioned grater.

Cut off the top and bottom of the squash and grate it lengthwise, using either the rough or fine side of the grater. Then place the squash in a colander and let it drain for half an hour. This removes the juice and makes the squash look more like pasta. Peel the sweet potato and grate it lengthwise and mix with the squash.

Cut black olives into halves and remove the pits.

Arrange the pasta on a plate, pour the pesto on top, and garnish with the halved olives.

You can easily make the dish without draining the grated squash, which makes it a quick and easy-to-prepare dinner.

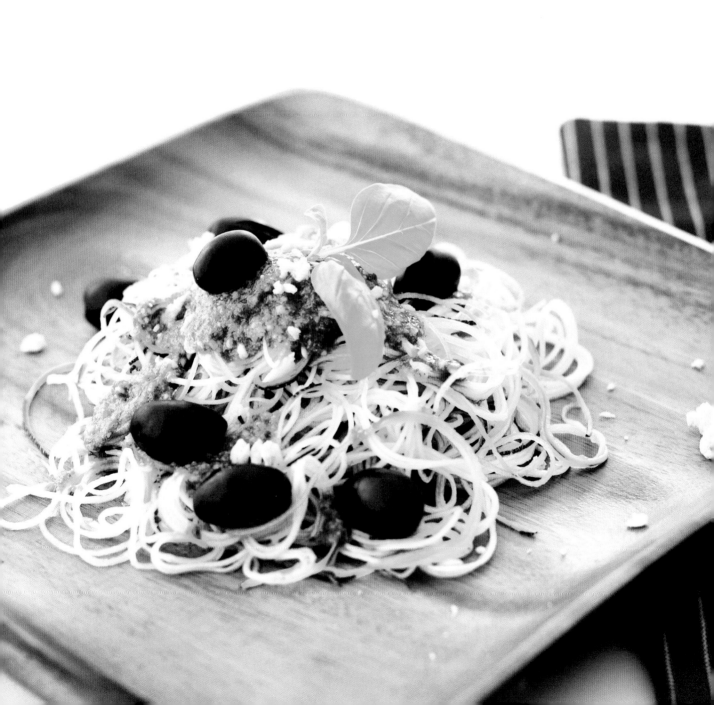

Pasta with Tomato Sauce

2 squash
Basic tomato sauce (p. 280)

2 tablespoons cashews, very finely chopped
1 handful basil leaves

Grate the squash lengthwise with a grater or use a spiral slicer.

Arrange the pasta on a plate and pour the tomato sauce over the pasta. Sprinkle with cashews and garnish with basil.

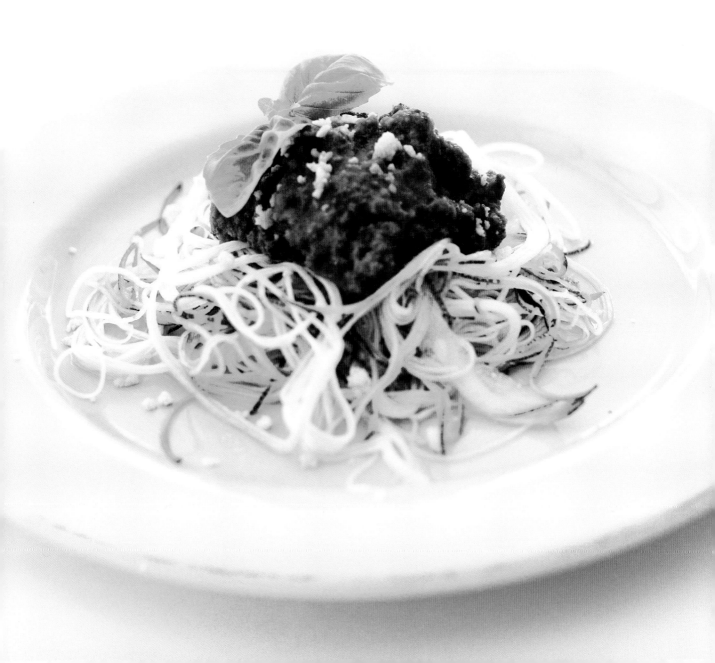

Pasta with Béchamel Sauce

2 sweet potatoes
10 cherry tomatoes
¾ cup (2 dls) peas
1 handful baby spinach
Béchamel sauce (p. 279)
2 tablespoons chopped parsley

Make the pasta by using the same procedure as for the pasta pesto. Slice the tomatoes into halves and take peas out of the pods (or thaw if they are frozen). Rinse spinach and remove the stems.

Arrange the spinach on a plate with the pasta and pour the béchamel sauce on top. Spread peas and tomatoes over the pasta and garnish with the chopped parsley.

Experiment with the kind of pasta you prefer. The three recipes above offer different ways of making the pasta. Find your favorite or combine them to make a multicolored pasta.

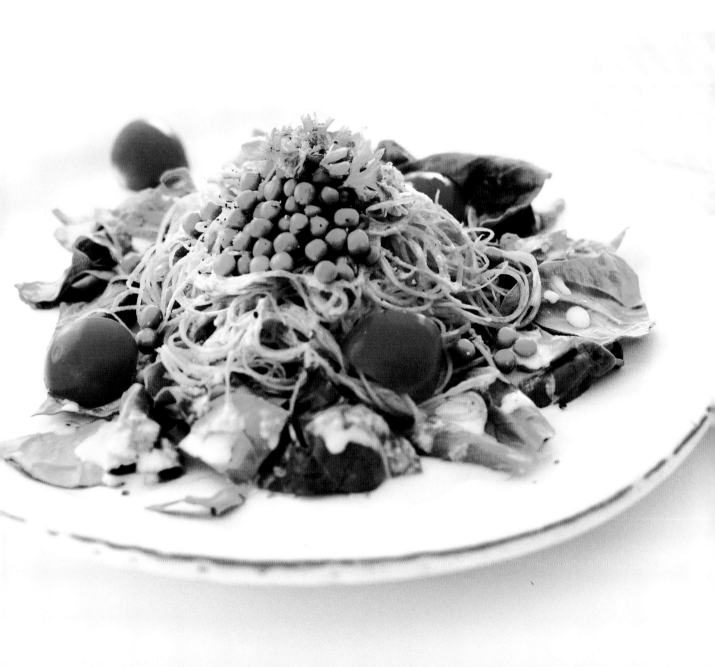

Walnut Meatloaf

¼ cup (½ dl) crushed linseed or hemp seed
Juice of 1 orange, or water
1¾ cup (4 dls) walnuts, soaked for 5 hours
1¾ cup (4 dls) mushrooms
2 carrots, grated
1 red onion
3 tablespoons avocado oil
2 teaspoons herbal salt
Pepper

Extra:
2 cloves garlic
2 stalks celery, chopped
½ teaspoon cayenne
2 tablespoons chopped parsley

Soak the linseed in orange juice (or water) for 5–10 minutes. Blend the walnuts, mushrooms, and onion in a food processor. Pour all other ingredients, including the orange juice, carrots, and seeds, into the mixture until it is well-combined.

If you want a plump meatloaf you can add the extra ingredients.

Optional: Serve on half a cabbage leaf with sliced radishes and béchamel sauce (p. 279).

You can also use this "minced meat" for lasagna (p. 120), or for pasta with tomato sauce (p. 280).

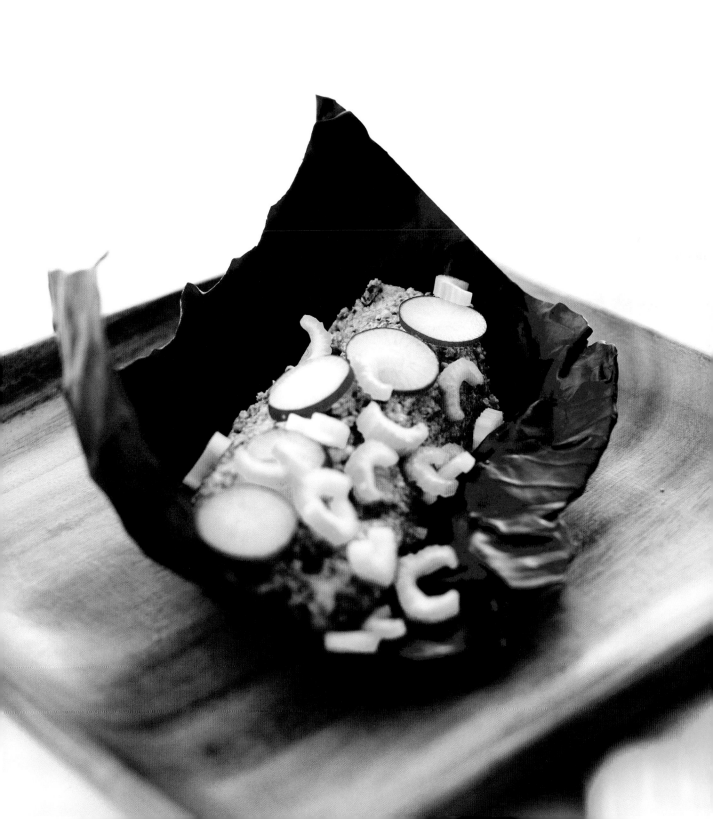

Chili sin Carne

¾ cup (150 g) dates
1 small shallot
½ cup (100 g) sun-dried tomatoes
1 teaspoon curry powder
1 chili pepper
¼ cup (½ dl) raw honey
3 cloves garlic, chopped
½ cup (1 dl) water
Cayenne pepper
Salt
1 shallot

1 green pepper
6 tomatoes
1¾ cups (400 g) germinated buckwheat, soaked 6 hours and sprouted 12–24 hours
1 corncob, kernels shaved off
¼ cup (½ dl) olive oil
Juice of 1 orange
½ tablespoon Bragg Liquid Aminos or Nama Shoyu

Blend dates, shallot, sun-dried tomatoes, curry, chili pepper, honey, and garlic with a little water. Add cayenne and salt to taste, and add the rest of the water to the mixture.

Chop the second shallot and dice the green pepper and the tomatoes. Mix all three ingredients in a bowl with the germinated buckwheat, corn, olive oil, orange juice, and soy sauce. Stir the sauce in with the other ingredients in a large bowl.

This dish tastes so fantastic that the first time I made it, I stuffed myself! I simply couldn't stop eating. This can be stored in the refrigerator for 3–5 days.

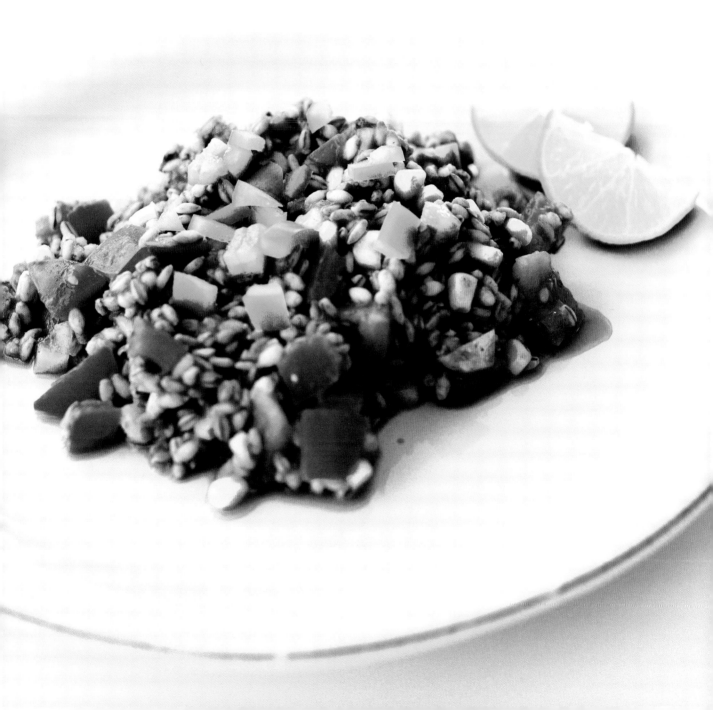

Raw Marinated Corn on the Cob

3 tablespoons olive oil

1–2 teaspoons coarse salt

4 ears of corn

Cayenne

Place a piece of aluminum foil large enough to wrap a corncob on a plate. Spread the oil on the aluminum foil and sprinkle with salt. Place a corncob on the foil and wrap it up. Repeat with the rest of the corncobs. Let them marinate for half an hour.

Unwrap the cobs and serve with a sprinkle of cayenne.

The fastest way to prepare this is to put oil in your palm and rub the corncobs, then sprinkle with salt and cayenne.

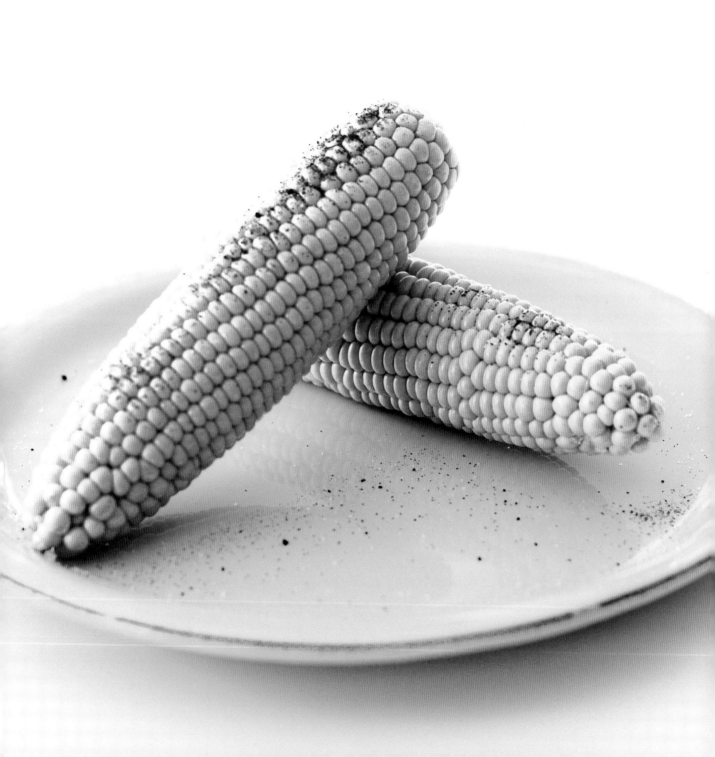

Look-alike Mashed Potatoes

1¼ cups (3 dls) cashews, soaked 1–2 hours
½ head of cauliflower
¼ cup (½ dl) olive oil
1–2 cloves garlic, minced
Water
Salt and pepper
Chili pepper

Garnish: 1 large beetroot
Parsley

Mushroom Cream

1¼ cups (3 dls) chopped Portobello mushrooms or a
    mix of mushrooms
1 clove garlic, minced
1 tablespoon olive oil
1 tablespoon Bragg Liquid Aminos, Nama Shoyu, or
    soy sauce
1 tablespoon water
1 teaspoon sage
½ teaspoon herbal salt
Pepper
1 handful fresh thyme

Look-alike Mashed Potatoes   Blend cashews, cauliflower, oil, and garlic in a food processor. Add water little by little until you have a creamy consistency. If you want extra finely mashed "potatoes," finish off by using a hand blender. Add salt, pepper, and chili pepper to taste.

Mushroom Cream   Blend all the mushroom cream ingredients in a food processor until you achieve a smooth consistency.

Peel and dice the beetroot.

Arrange the look-alike mashed potatoes on a plate. Pour the mushroom cream on top and garnish with the diced beetroot and parsley.

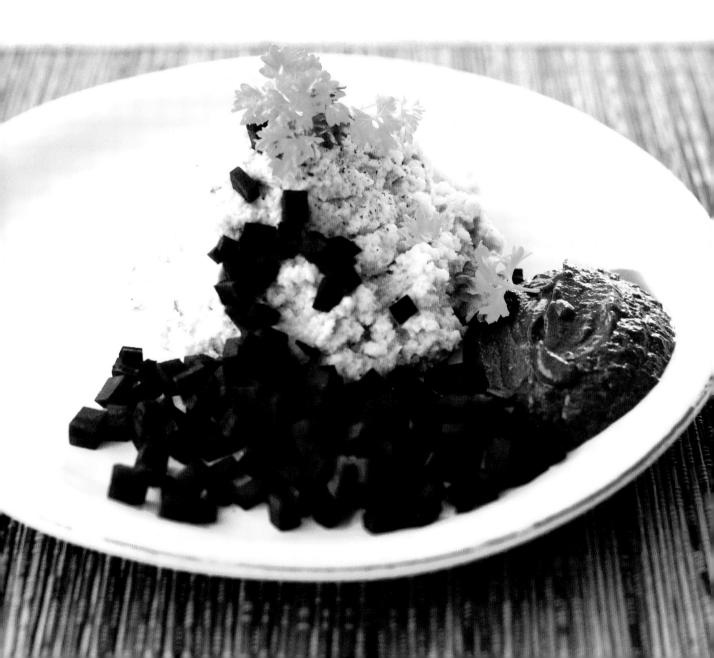

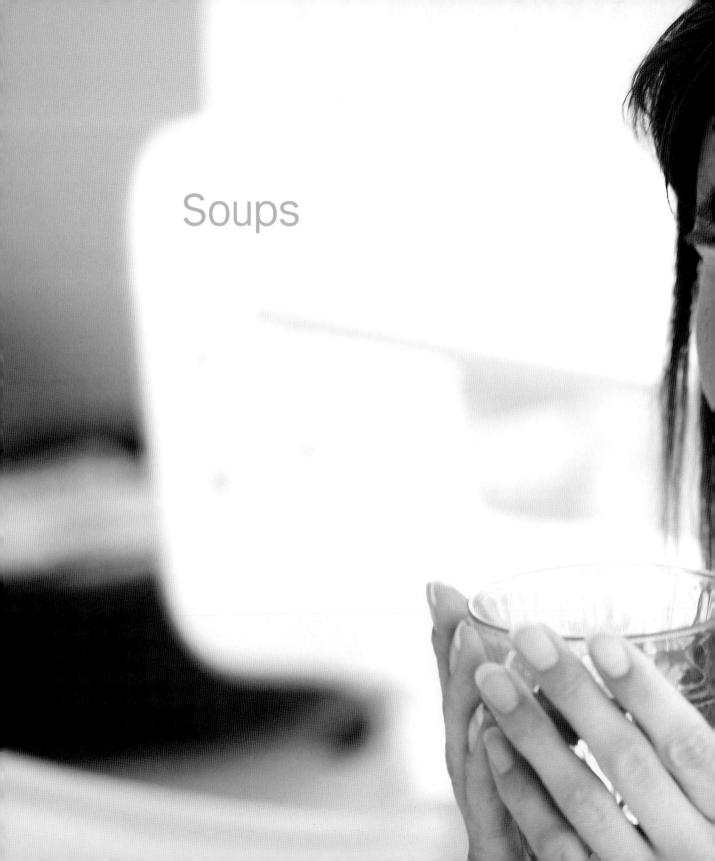

Soups

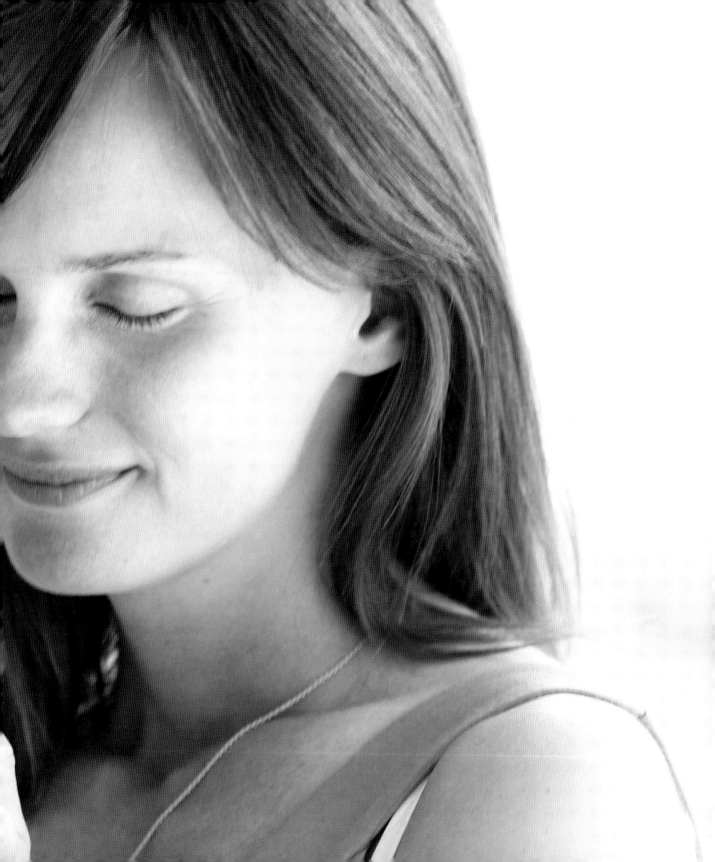

Soups are quick and easy to make, and because nutrients in liquid form are more easily absorbed, your body does not need to use energy to break down the food. It's a terrific way of getting an energy kick.

Pineapple and Cucumber Soup

2 cucumbers
1 scallion
1 pineapple
1 small chili pepper
Salt and pepper

4 tablespoons avocado oil
1 tablespoon lime juice

½ cup (1 dl) fresh chopped herbs (optional)

Peel the cucumbers and cut them into small pieces. Chop the scallion. Peel and core the pineapple and cut it into slices. Blend ¾ pineapple and ¾ cucumber, ¾ scallion, avocado, lime juice, and half the chili pepper (without seeds). Add extra chili pepper, salt, and pepper to taste.

Garnish with the remaining pineapple, cucumber, and scallion, then serve.

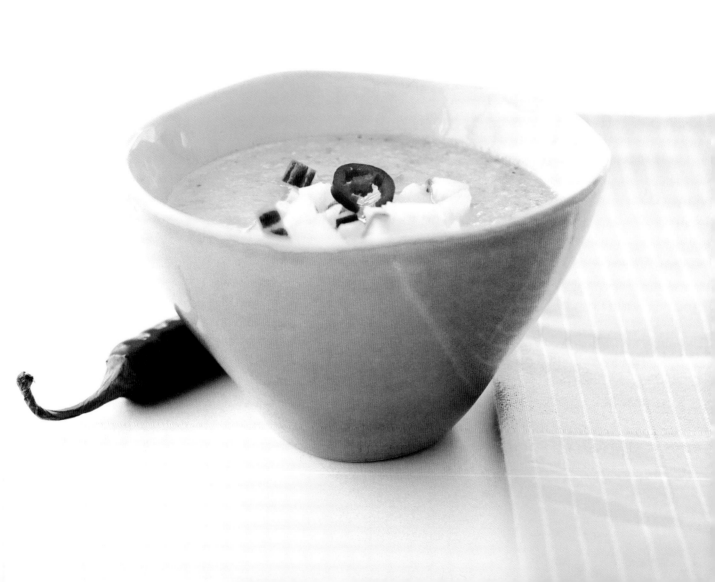

Gazpacho

8 tomatoes
1 cucumber
2 cups (5 dls) watermelon (or other melon)
1 scallion
2 cloves garlic, minced
Cayenne pepper (or chili or Tabasco sauce)
2 tablespoons lime juice
Salt and pepper

Garnish: cilantro

Chop the tomatoes, cucumber, watermelon, and scallion into small pieces. Mix half of them in a blender with the garlic, cayenne, and lime juice. Combine the rest of the chopped vegetables with the blended mixture and add extra cayenne, salt, and pepper to taste.

Garnish with fresh cilantro.

Try serving with frozen strawberries or ice cubes.

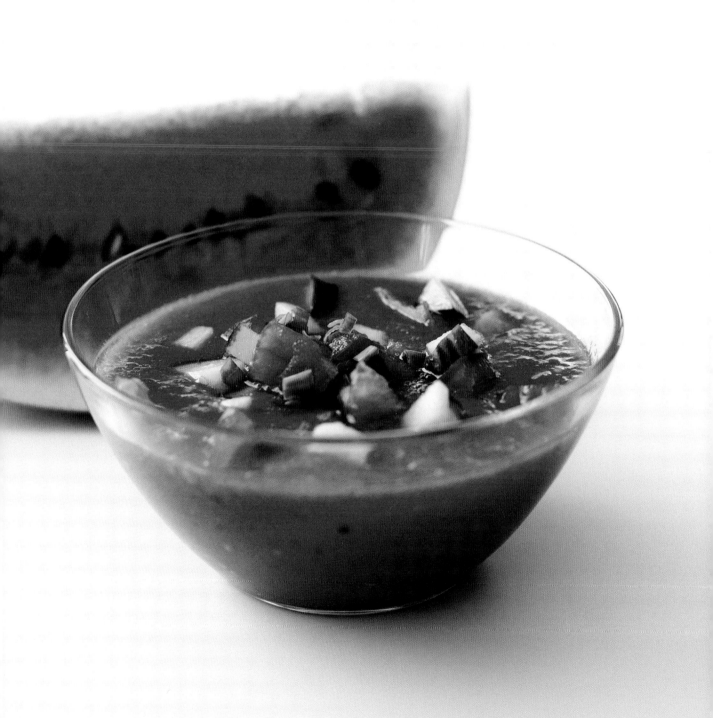

Pea Soup

1 pint (½ l) water
¾ cup (150 g) almonds
1¾ cups (450 g) peas

1 avocado
1 small handful fresh mint
Salt and pepper
Freshly grated nutmeg

First make the almond milk (p. 270). Then mix with peas, avocado, and half the mint, and blend. Add salt, pepper, and freshly grated nutmeg to taste. Garnish with mint and serve.

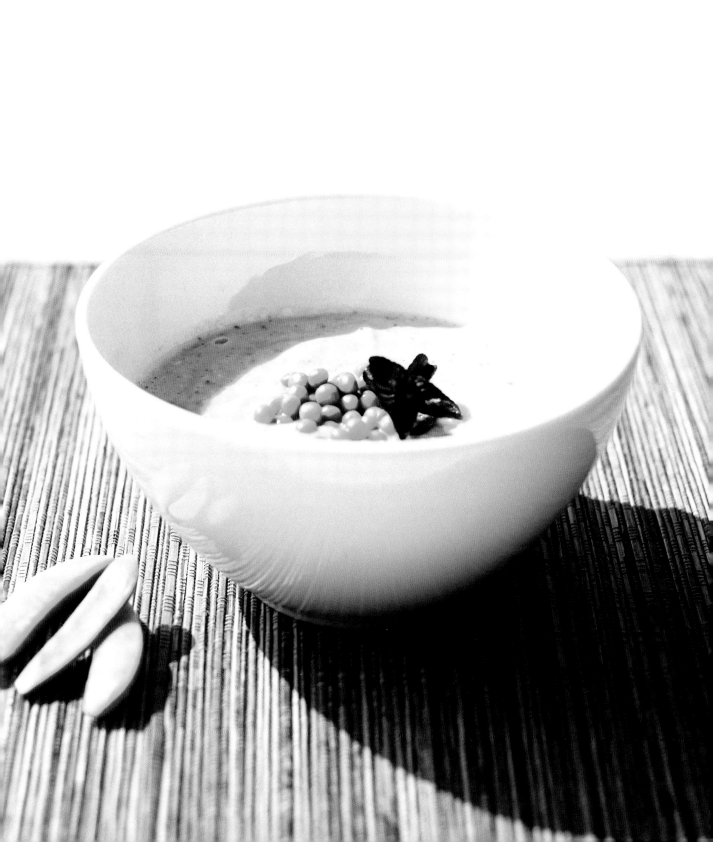

Light and Fluffy Pepper Bisque

2 bell peppers
¾ cup (2 dls) cashew nut milk (p. 272)
1 cucumber
Juice of ½ orange
4 tablespoons sesame oil or avocado oil
¼ teaspoon cayenne
Salt to taste

Garnish: Oil
Freshly ground black pepper

Remove stems, seeds, and membranes from the bell peppers. Chop the peppers and blend with the remaining ingredients in a blender until light and fluffy. Serve in a bowl and garnish with a circle of oil and freshly ground black pepper.

You can substitute dulse or kelp for the salt. Both dulse and kelp are rich in iodine and other minerals.

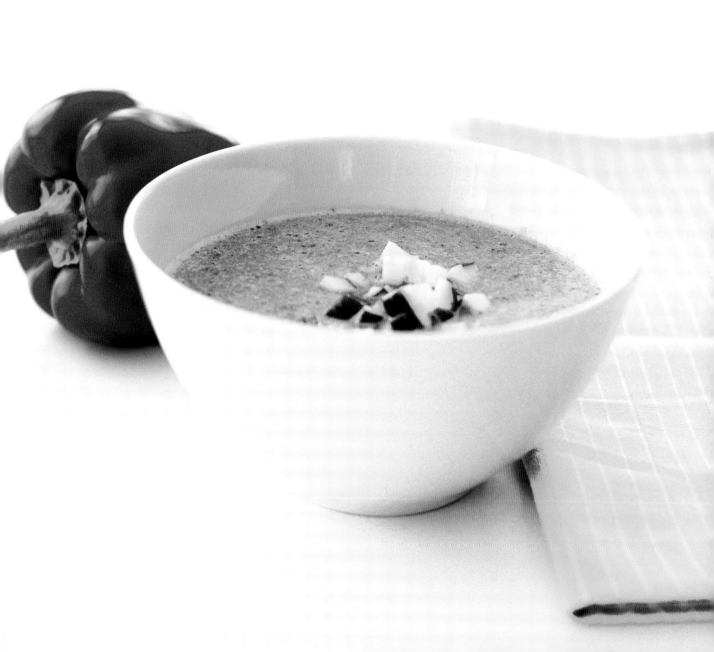

Corn Chowder

3⅓ cups (8 dls) almond milk (p. 270)
5 corncobs, kernels shaved off
1 avocado
Salt

First make the almond milk, then mix with corn and avocado and blend. Add salt to taste.

For those who prefer a slightly stronger taste, the following can be added:

2 scallions
3 tablespoons avocado oil
1 clove garlic
Jalapeño and lemon juice to taste

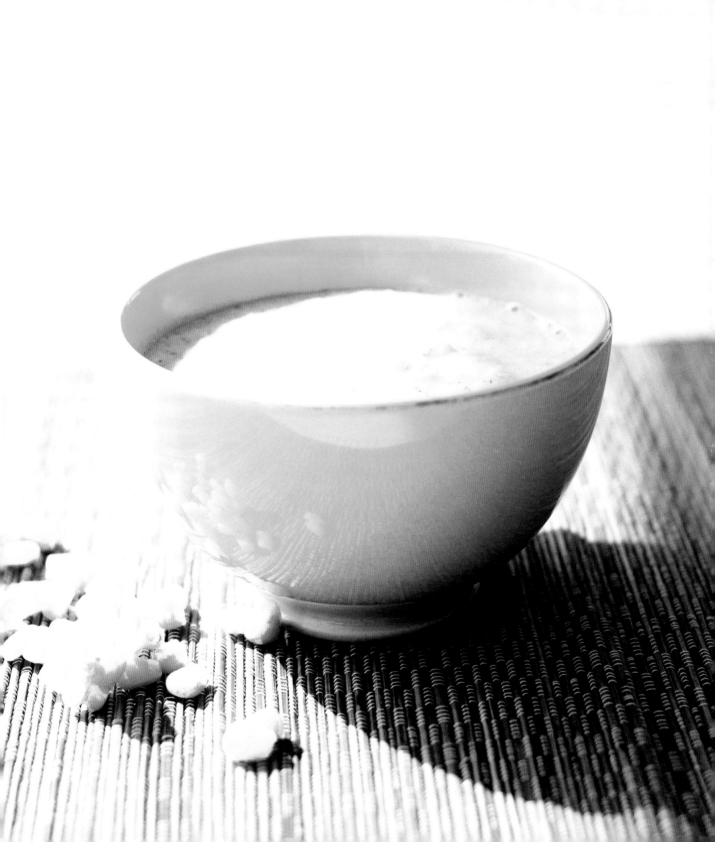

Simple Cucumber Soup

1 avocado
1 cucumber, sliced
Juice of 1 lime
4 tablespoons dill (or thyme)
Salt
Water
1 tablespoon tahini

Garnish: 1 tablespoon olive oil

Blend all ingredients except for a couple of cucumber slices, the oil, and some dill.

Serve in a bowl and garnish with cucumber slices, oil, and dill.

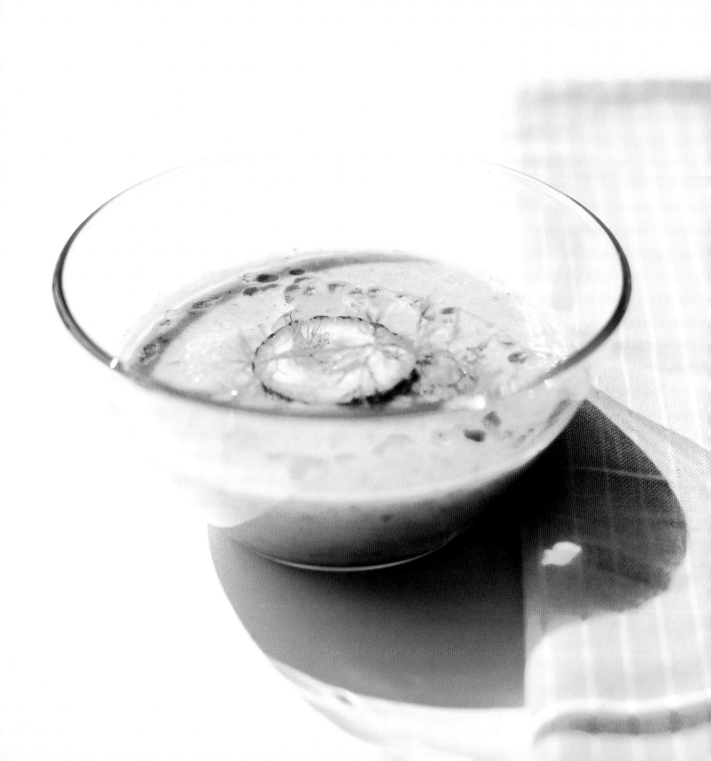

Fantastic Celery Soup

¾ cup (220 g) cashews, soaked 3 hours
3⅓ cups (8 dls) water
½ celeriac (600 g)
2 apples
6 tablespoons olive oil
¾ cup (1½ dls) chives, chopped
2 tablespoons coconut oil
1 teaspoon lime juice
1 teaspoon honey
1 teaspoon paprika powder
Salt and pepper

Garnish: 1 tablespoon grated lemon zest

Blend nuts and 1¾ cups (4 dls) water to a milky consistency. Pour the milk into a food processor. Peel the celery, cut it in large pieces, and add to the food processor. Core the apples and put ¾ of them in the food processor. Dice the rest of the apple and save for garnish. (If you're not using it right away, you can sprinkle the apple with lemon juice so it doesn't turn brown). Save ¼ cup (½ dl) of the chives for garnish. Add the rest of the ingredients to the food processor and blend until the mixture is a creamy soup. Add paprika, salt, and pepper to taste.

Serve in bowls and garnish with paprika, apple, chives, and lemon zest.

Here we use a solid Danish vegetable, which is affordable and loaded with healthy dietary fiber. I must admit that I am usually not a big fan of the taste of celery, but this soup is so delicious that I added raisins to the leftovers and ate it for breakfast the first time I made it.

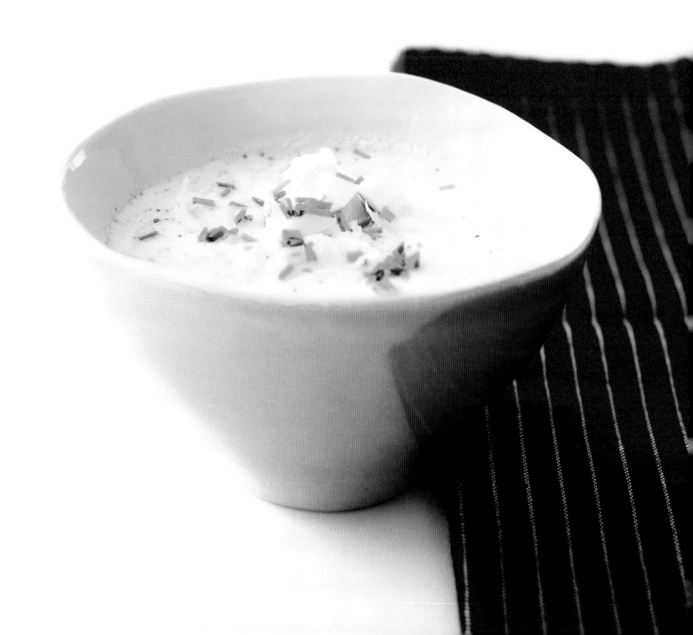

Beetroot Soup

2–3 beetroots
1 tablespoon olive oil
1 pinch of salt
1 pinch of vanilla powder (or more to make the soup taste more like a dessert)
Fresh ginger (optional, in whatever quantity you enjoy)
Water (enough to barely cover the beetroots)

Fresh mint

Peel the beetroots and cut into large dices. Mix all the ingredients in a food processor and blend until the consistency is just the way you like it. Season the soup. Garnish with mint and serve.

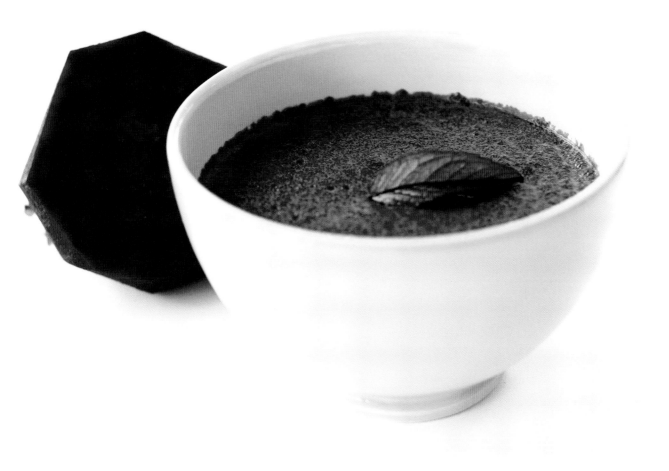

Easy Tomato Soup

1 coconut (¼ of the coconut meat, all of the milk)
8 tomatoes
4 sun-dried tomatoes
2–3 tablespoons ginger, finely chopped
1 clove garlic, minced
½ chili pepper, chopped

Herbal salt
Freshly ground black pepper

Split the coconut and pour the coconut milk into a blender. Remove ¼ of the coconut meat from the shell, chop it into smaller pieces, and mix it with the milk. Chop all the fresh tomatoes and three of the sun-dried tomatoes and mix with coconut, ginger, chili pepper, and garlic. Blend until you have a soft and creamy soup. Season with herbal salt and pepper.

Cut one sun-dried tomato into thin slices and use it as garnish.

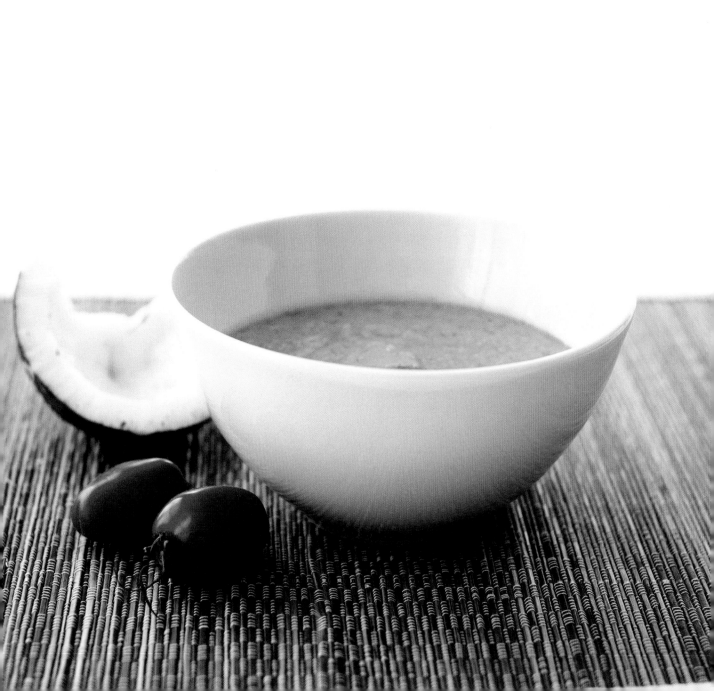

Carrot Soup

5 carrots
¼ teaspoon cayenne
1 tablespoon olive oil
1 pinch of salt
1 pinch of vanilla powder
Fresh ginger to taste
Water (enough to barely cover the carrots)

Peel the carrots and cut into large pieces. Add all the ingredients to a food processor and blend until the consistency is just the way you like it. Season the soup and serve.

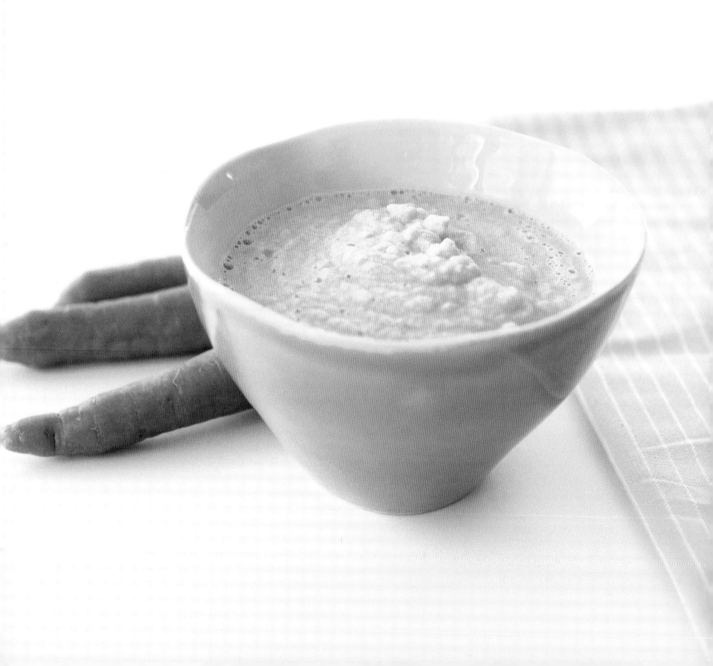

Shiitake and Seaweed Soup

2 tablespoons (30 g) arame seaweed

1 handful shiitake mushrooms

1 scallion, finely chopped

1¾ cups (4 dls) almond milk (p. 270)

3 tablespoons sesame or avocado oil

1 tablespoon Bragg Liquid Aminos or Nama Shoyu

Herbal salt

1 teaspoon raw cacao

Soak the seaweed in water until it is soft but still springy. Remove stalks from the mushrooms and cut the mushrooms into small pieces. Blend half of the mushrooms, seaweed, and scallion with the almond milk, oil, raw cacao, and soy sauce. Add herbal salt to taste. Pour the soup into bowls and use the rest of the mushrooms, scallion, and seaweed to form a variety of shapes and place them in the middle of the soup. Be creative!

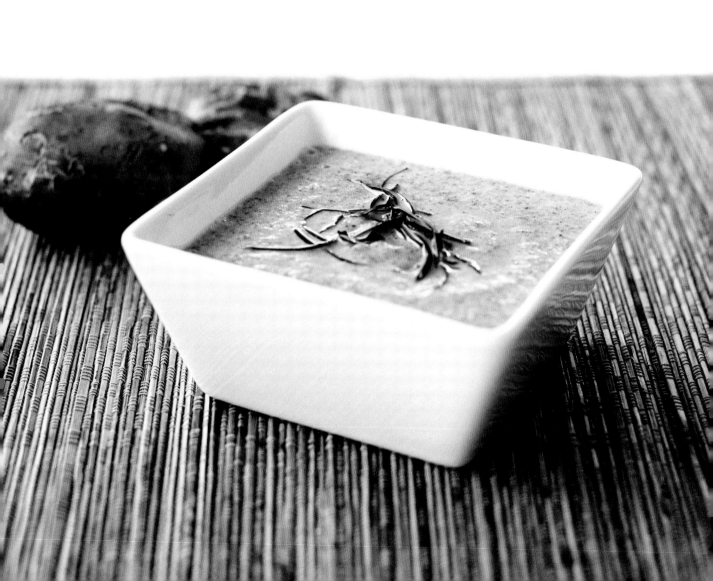

Broccoli Soup

2½ cups (6 dls) water
1 cup (200 g) almonds
1 teaspoon honey
¾ head of broccoli
1 ripe avocado
1 clove garlic
2 tablespoons avocado oil
¼ red onion
Salt and pepper
½ teaspoon caraway seeds

Blend water, almonds, and honey until milky. Chop the broccoli, avocado, garlic, and onion and blend in a food processor or blender and blend until the consistency is just the way you like it. Add salt, pepper, and caraway seeds to taste.

If you want a silk-like soup, pour it through a strainer.

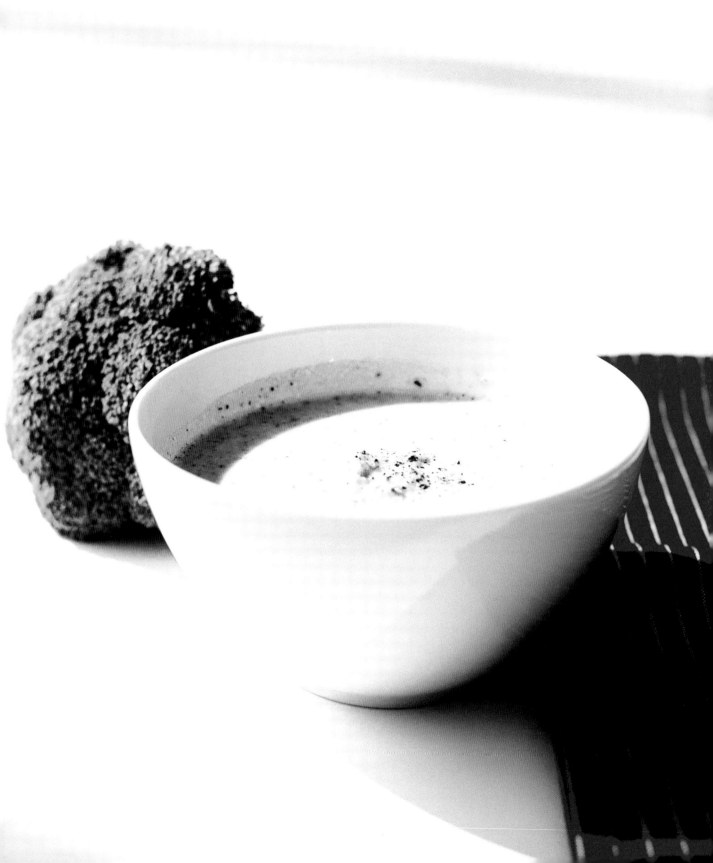

Asparagus Soup

2 radishes
1–2 bunches of green or white asparagus
1 scallion
¼ cup (50 g) kale, stems removed
1 stalk celery
1 handful fresh thyme and rosemary
½ teaspoon raw honey
1 avocado, peeled and pit removed
1¼ cups (3 dls) water
Salt

Cut the radishes into thin slices and set them aside for garnishing with a bit of the fresh herbs. Chop the asparagus, scallion, kale, and celery into small pieces and mix with the rest of the ingredients in a blender. Blend until you have a creamy soup. Strain the soup and garnish with fresh herbs and radishes.

If you prefer a less bitter soup, you can remove the heads of the asparagus and use them for something else.

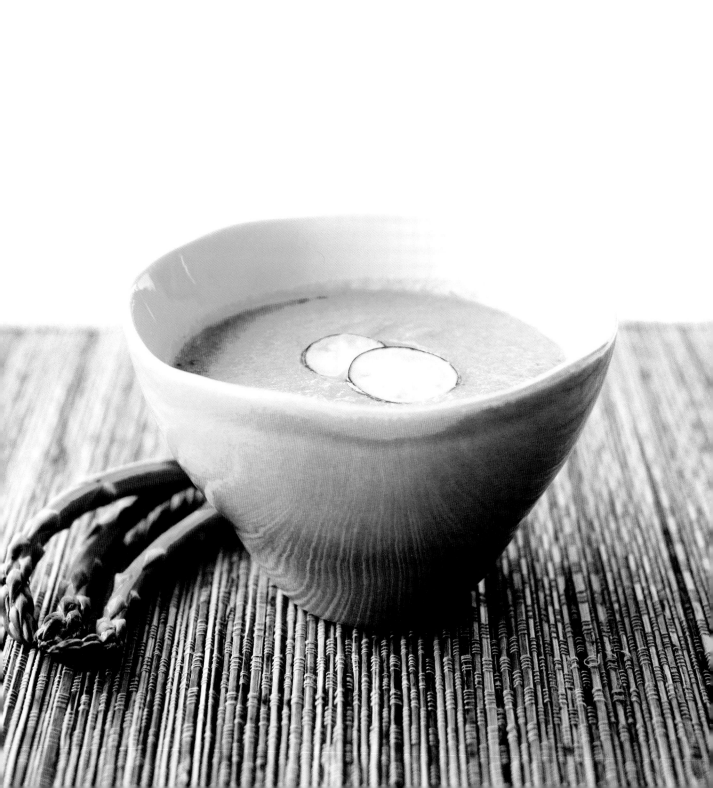

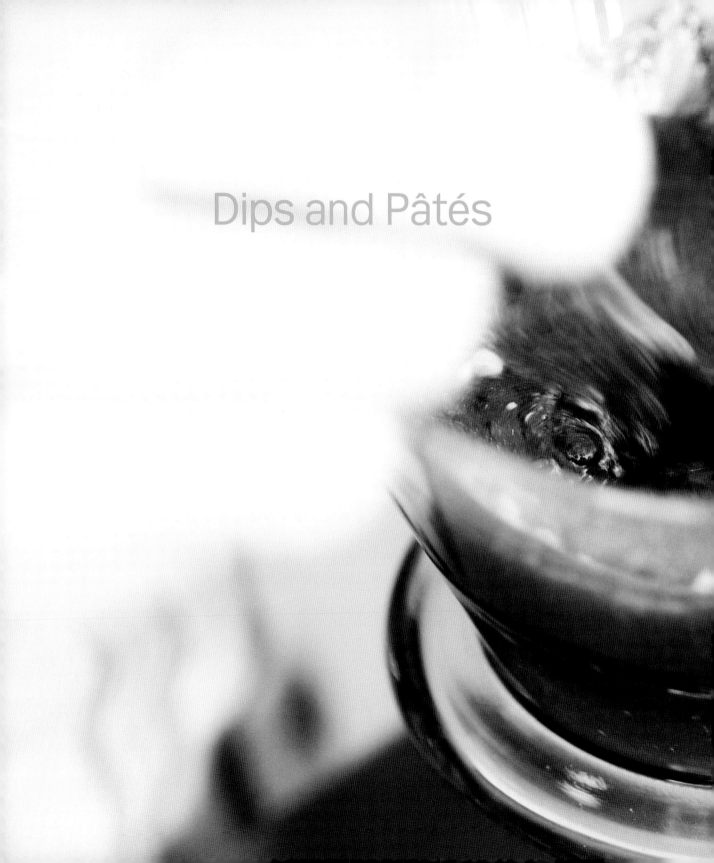

Dips and Pâtés

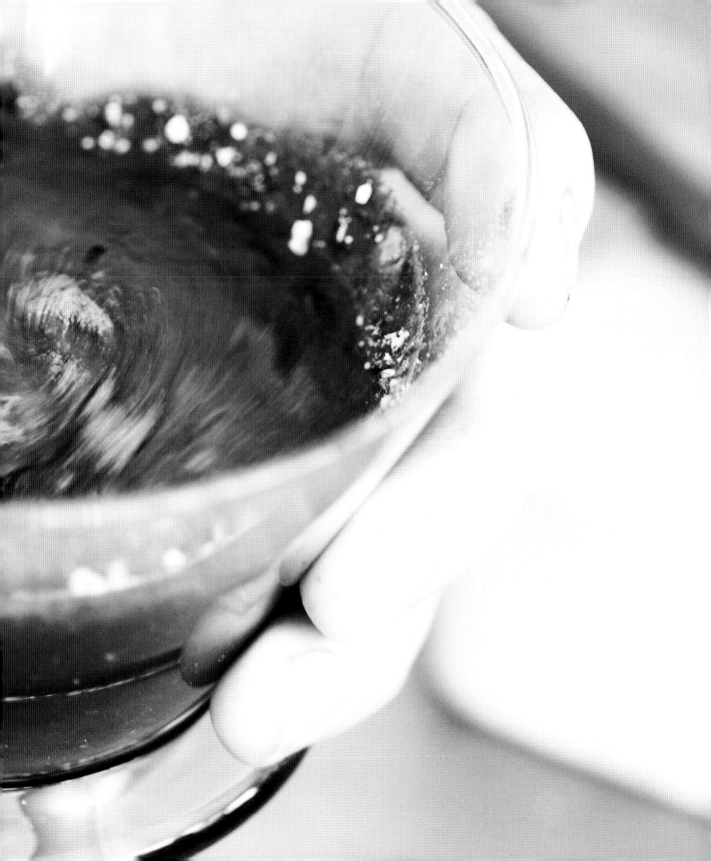

Too-Easy-to-Be-Real Cashew Butter

1¾ cups (400 g) cashews or mixed nuts

Put all the nuts into a food processor and blend until the mixture forms a moist ball. This takes a while, so beware of not overheating the food processor; stop the machine every couple minutes, scraping down the sides of the bowl from time to time.

You can add some oil if you use almonds, as the ball may become too dry.

The nut butter lasts longer if you don't use oil.

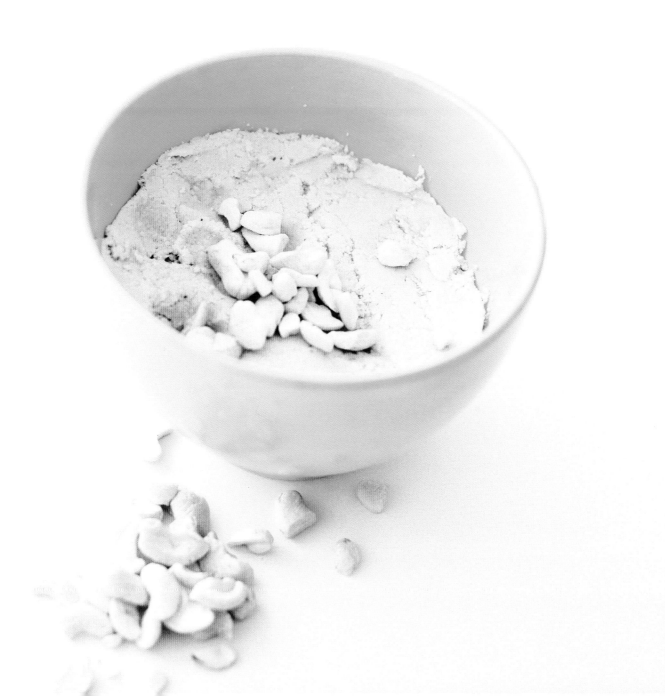

2 cucumbers
2 teaspoons salt
2–3 cloves minced garlic
3⅓ cups (8 dls) raw yogurt (p. 52)
2 tablespoons olive oil

Garnish:
Olives
Olive oil
Cucumber slices

Cut the cucumbers in half and remove the seeds. Grate the cucumbers, put them into a strainer, and sprinkle with salt. Let them drain and then use your hands to press the rest of the juice from the cucumber.

Mix garlic, raw yogurt, and olive oil together and add the drained grated cucumber.

Arrange on a dish with olives, olive oil, and slices of cucumber.

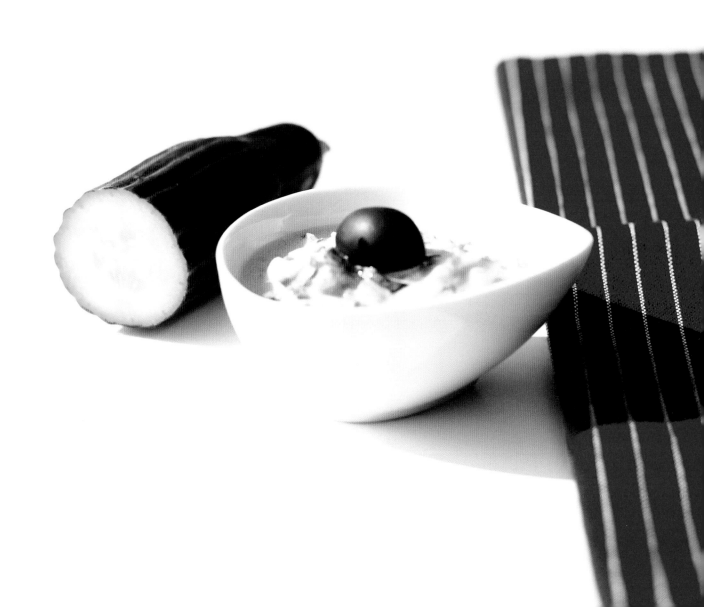

Mayonnaise

¾ cup (2 dls) nut milk
3 tablespoons avocado
1½ tablespoons apple cider vinegar
1 teaspoon salt
¾ cup (2 dls) cold-pressed grapeseed oil or sunflower oil

Blend the nut milk, avocado, vinegar, and salt with a hand blender, then slowly pour the oil into the mixture while continuing to blend.

Before using the mayonnaise, put it in the refrigerator for a couple of hours until it thickens. You can also adjust the thickness by adding more avocado or vinegar.

For a different taste, you can make the nut milk with cucumber instead of water.

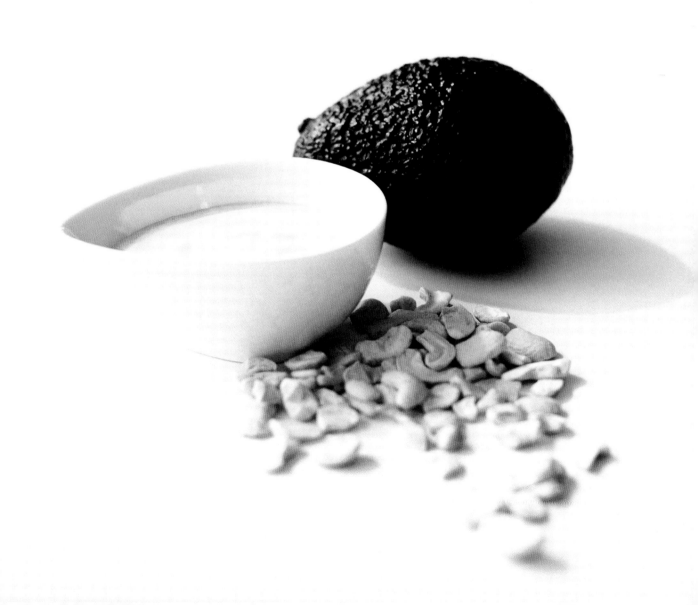

Easy Hummus Made with Sunflower Seeds

2 cups (5 dls) sunflower seeds, soaked for 2 hours
½ cup (1 dl) water
Juice of 1 lemon
2 cloves garlic, minced
½ cup (1 dl) olive oil or sesame oil
1 teaspoon salt
1 teaspoon ground cumin
2 tablespoons tahini (optional)

Hummus

2 cups (5 dls) sprouted mung beans or chickpeas
⅓ cup (¾ dl) tahini
½ red onion, chopped
2–4 cloves garlic, minced
¾ cup (1½ dls) olive oil
Juice of 1 lemon
1 teaspoon ground cumin
1 teaspoon salt

Garnish:
1 handful chopped parsley

Easy Hummus Made with Sunflower Seeds Mix all the ingredients together in a blender. You can adjust the consistency by using more or less oil and water. This is a quick way to prepare delicious hummus.

Hummus Soak the mung beans or chickpeas overnight and let them sprout for a couple of days. Rinse twice a day. Use a food processor or blender to mix all the ingredients. I prefer a chunky consistency but you can blend the hummus finely if you prefer it that way.

You can change the color of the hummus by adding black olives, grated carrots, or red bell peppers. You can substitute the tahini with sesame oil if you prefer.

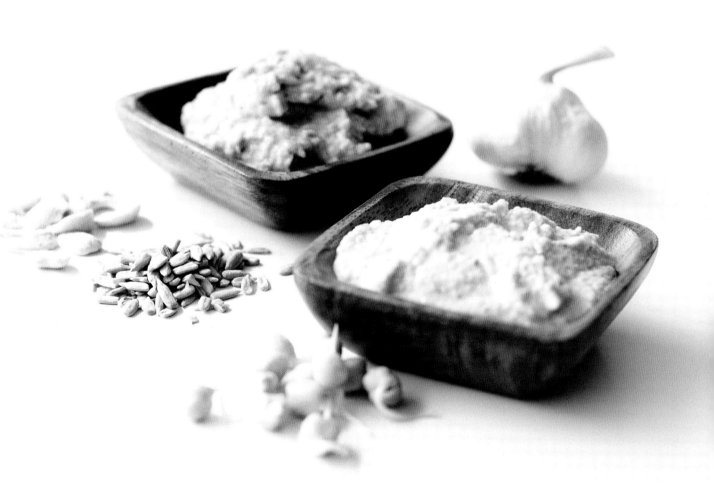

Raw Tahini

½ cup (1 dl) sesame seeds
¼ cup (½ dl) sesame oil
Salt

Grind the seeds in a coffee grinder until they are the consistency of flour or are finely chopped. Blend the crushed seeds and oil together with a hand blender, gradually adding the oil a little at a time. Season with salt.

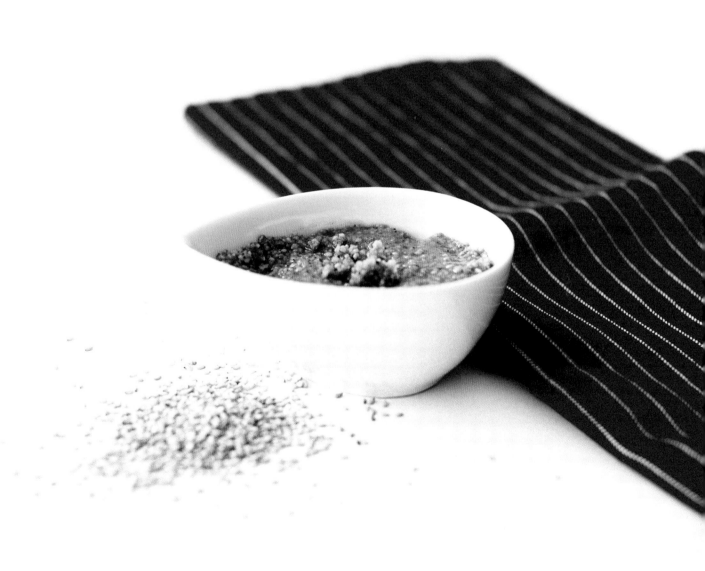

Olive Tapenade

½ cup (1 dl) olive oil
3 tablespoons chopped parsley
3 tablespoons chopped basil
1 clove garlic, chopped
1 tablespoon lemon juice
Salt and pepper
12 olives, pitted

Blend all the ingredients except the olives together until the mixture is creamy. Add the pitted olives and blend until you can only see small pieces of olive.

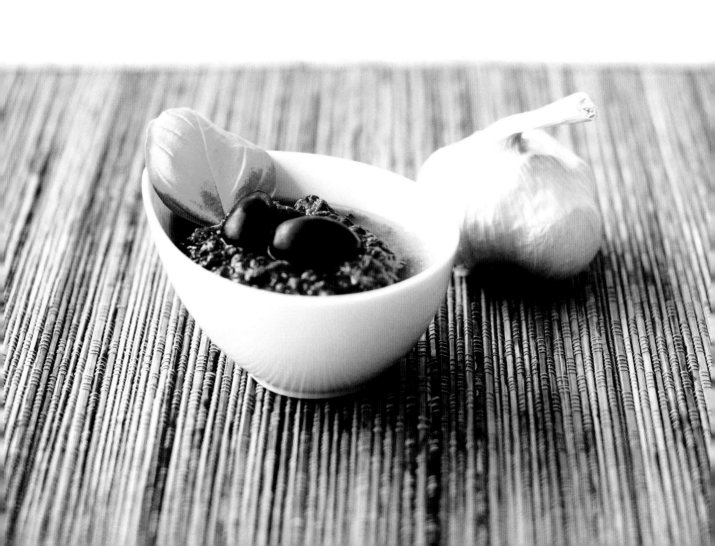

Jerusalem Artichoke Purée

2 cups (500 g) Jerusalem artichoke
1 shallot
½ cup (1 dl) "You Just Might Think It's Crème Fraîche" (p. 262)
¼ cup (½ dl) avocado oil
1 tablespoon lemon juice
1 teaspoon herbal salt
Pepper

Peel the Jerusalem artichokes and shallot and chop them into small pieces. Mix with all other ingredients in a blender. Add water if necessary, and salt and pepper to taste.

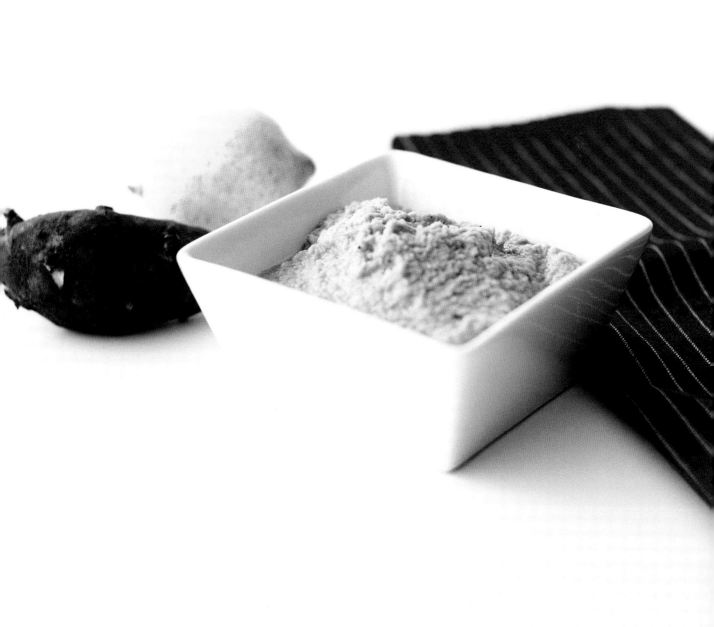

Pesto

1¼ cup (3 dls) olive oil

½ cup (1 dl) cashews

1 bunch of fresh basil (or parsley)

2 cloves garlic, minced

1 tablespoon salt

Mix all the ingredients in a blender.

There is no need to buy pesto; it is so easy to make. You can experiment until you have your favorite flavor. For a taste closer to the authentic taste of pesto, substitute avocado oil for the olive oil.

Sun-dried Tomato Pesto

¾ cup (2 dls) olive oil

½ cup (1 dl) cashews

½ cup (1 dl) sun-dried tomatoes (soaked 2 hours)

2 cloves garlic

2 teaspoons lemon juice

2 tablespoons fresh herbs

¼ teaspoon cayenne

Salt and pepper

Blend all the ingredients in a blender. (I use cashews instead of pine nuts for this pesto, since I'm not much for the taste of raw pine nuts. I think cashews have the right taste and consistency.)

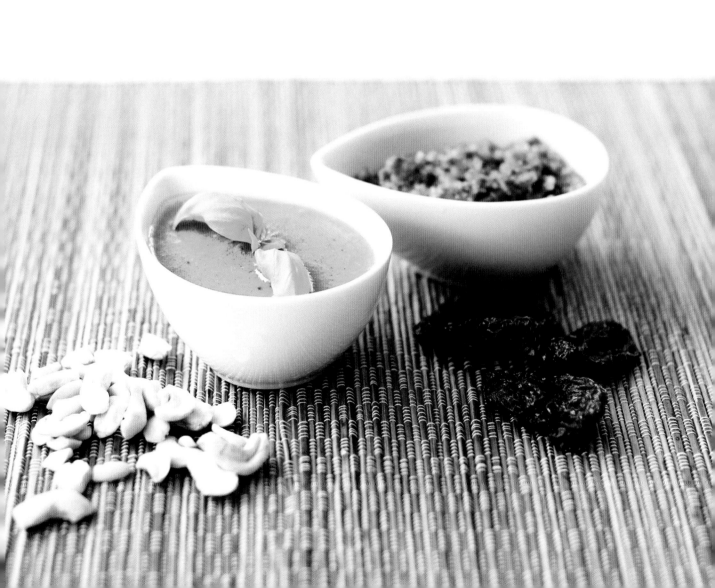

Easy Guacamole

2 ripe avocados
1 tablespoon lime juice
2 teaspoons cumin powder
¼ teaspoon cayenne pepper
1 teaspoon herbal salt

Remove skin and pit from the avocados. Combine all the ingredients until creamy but still chunky.

The recipe can be expanded with:
½ chopped tomato
1 clove garlic, minced
½ chopped red onion
Fresh coriander

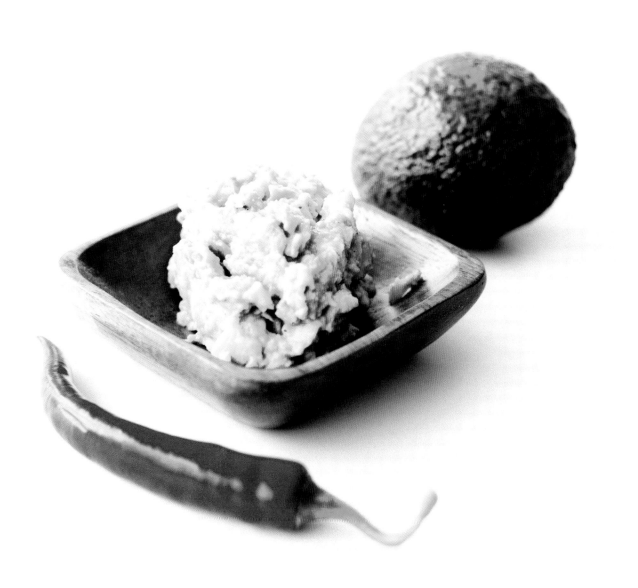

Look-alike Salmon Pâté

1 cup (250 g) walnuts, soaked 6 hours
1 stalk celery
1 large red bell pepper
1 shallot
½–1 teaspoon salt

Peel the shallot and chop it together with the celery and the red bell pepper. Mix all the ingredients in a food processor and blend until the consistency is like pâté.

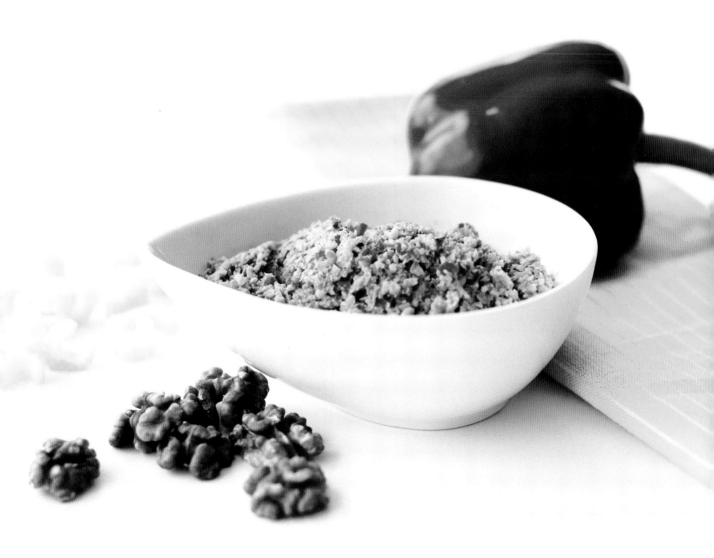

Pea Pâté

¾ cup (150 g) walnuts, soaked 6–8 hours
1½ cups (350 g) peas
½ teaspoon salt
2 tablespoons (25 g) ginger (can be crushed in a garlic press)
1 pinch of cayenne pepper (optional)

Drain walnuts and mix all the ingredients in a food processor. Blend until creamy. Add extra salt and ginger to taste.

Red Cabbage Crunch

½ cup (100 g) pumpkin seeds, soaked 6 hours
1 cup (200 g) red cabbage, chopped
5 dates, pitted
¼ red onion or 1 shallot
Juice of 1 orange (optional)

Drain the pumpkin seeds and mix all the ingredients in a food processor until well combined.

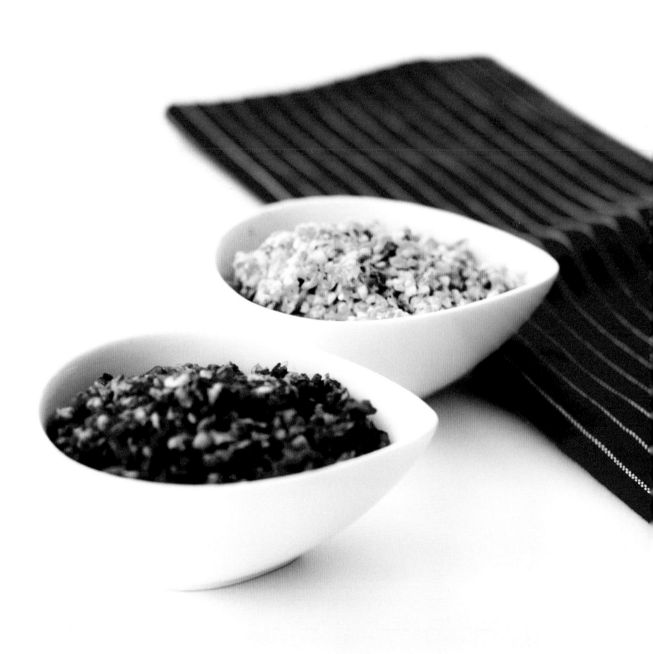

Sunflower Pâté

1½ cups (300 g) sunflower seeds, soaked 8–12 hours
Juice of 1 lime
2–3 shallots, chopped
4–6 tablespoons chopped parsley
2–3 cloves garlic, minced
½ teaspoon cayenne (or more)
1 handful fresh basil
2 teaspoons ground cumin
2 teaspoons salt

Lettuce
Avocado
Cherry tomatoes

Mix all the ingredients in a food processor and blend until the pâté is creamy and delicious.

Serve on a few leaves of lettuce garnished with tomatoes and avocado.

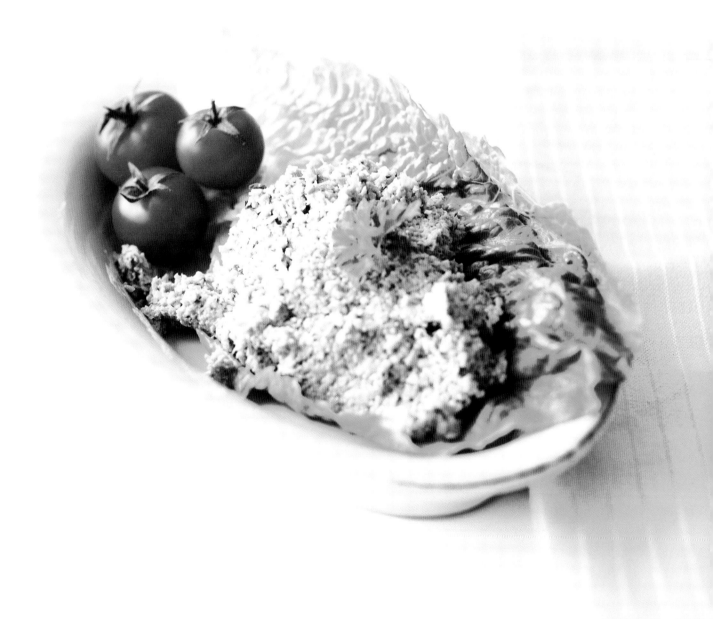

Dill Cream Cheese

½–¾ cup (1–2 dls) water
¾ cup (2 dls) cashews, soaked at least 2 hours
½ cup (1 dl) finely chopped dill
1 tablespoon herbal salt
1 pinch of cayenne pepper

Pour half of the water into the blender and slowly add the cashews, alternately pouring more water and blending. Add cashews until you have a thick mass. Add more water if needed. When the mixture looks like cream cheese, add the rest of the ingredients and mix.

Dill can be replaced by other herbs, curry powder, or paprika.

Sun-dried Tomato Cream Cheese

¾ cup (2 dls) macadamia nuts, soaked overnight
½–¾ cup (1–2 dls) water
⅓ cup (¾ dl) sun-dried tomatoes, soaked 1–2 hours
1 tablespoon olive oil
½ tablespoon apple cider vinegar
½–1 teaspoon herbal salt
½ teaspoon paprika powder

Pour half of the water into the blender and slowly add the macadamia nuts, alternately pouring more water and blending. Add macadamia nuts until you have a thick mass. Add more water if needed. When the mixture looks like cream cheese, add the rest of the ingredients and mix.

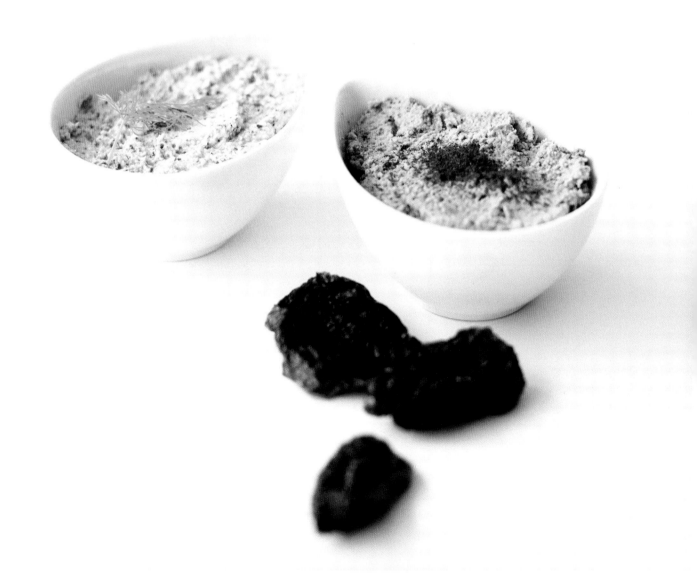

Paprika Dip

1 red bell pepper
1 green bell pepper
1 avocado
¾ cup (2 dls) finely chopped broccoli
1 tablespoon onion, chopped
1 teaspoon cumin

1 teaspoon salt
1 pinch of cayenne pepper

Chop the bell peppers into smaller chunks and add them to the blender (or use a hand blender) together with the avocado meat and the rest of the ingredients. Season with spices. If you want the dip to be thinner, add a little water.

Sour Cream and Onion Dip

¾ cup (2 dls) macadamia nuts or cashews
⅓ cup (¾ dl) water
½ cup (1 dl) chopped onion
1 tablespoon apple cider vinegar
½ teaspoon salt

Mix all the ingredients in a blender. Add a little water to make sure it gets thick and creamy.

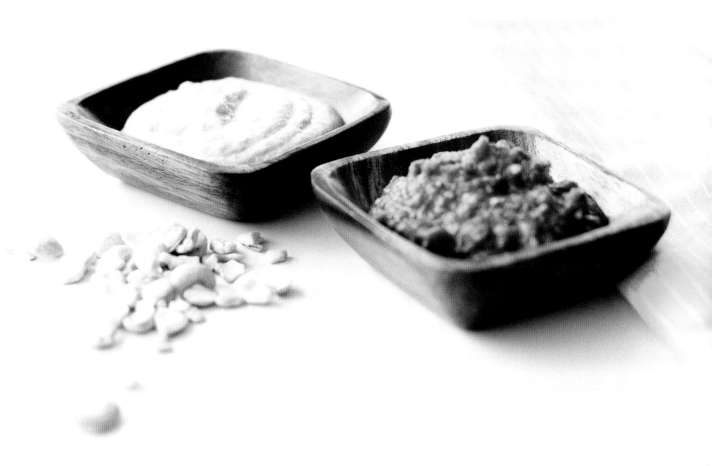

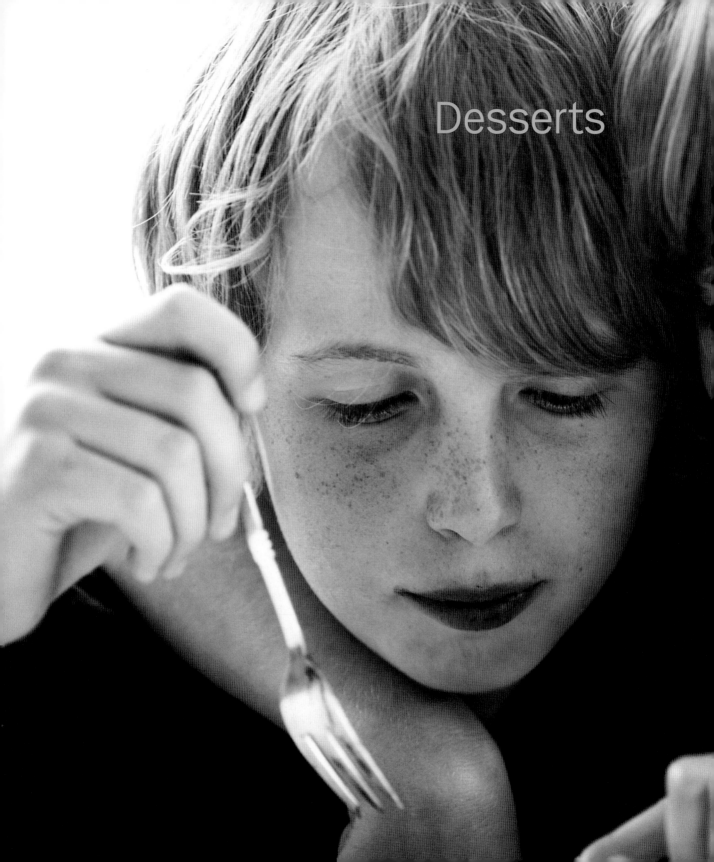

Desserts

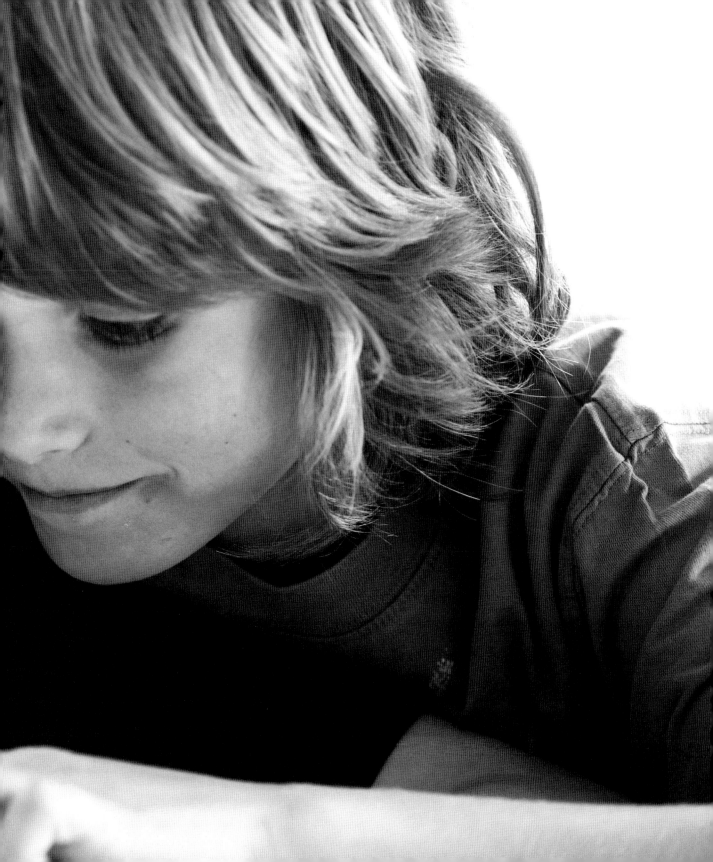

This is pure wonderland. Eat as many desserts as you want to. They are all extremely healthy.

Cashew-Stracciatella Ice Cream

2½ cups (6 dls) cashews
½ cup (1 dl) agave nectar
¾–1¼ cups (2–3 dls) water
1 teaspoon vanilla
1–2 tablespoons coconut oil (optional)
¼ cup (½ dl) hazelnuts
3 tablespoons raw cacao nibs

Blend the cashews in a food processor until you have nut butter. Add agave nectar, water, and vanilla and mix. Chop the hazelnuts and carefully mix the nuts and cacao nibs into the mass. Put it in the freezer, and after a couple of hours you will have the most delicious ice cream.

For a different taste, try replacing cashews with hazelnut butter or almond butter.

This is my favorite ice cream. If I am home alone, I make one portion for myself. What self-indulgence!

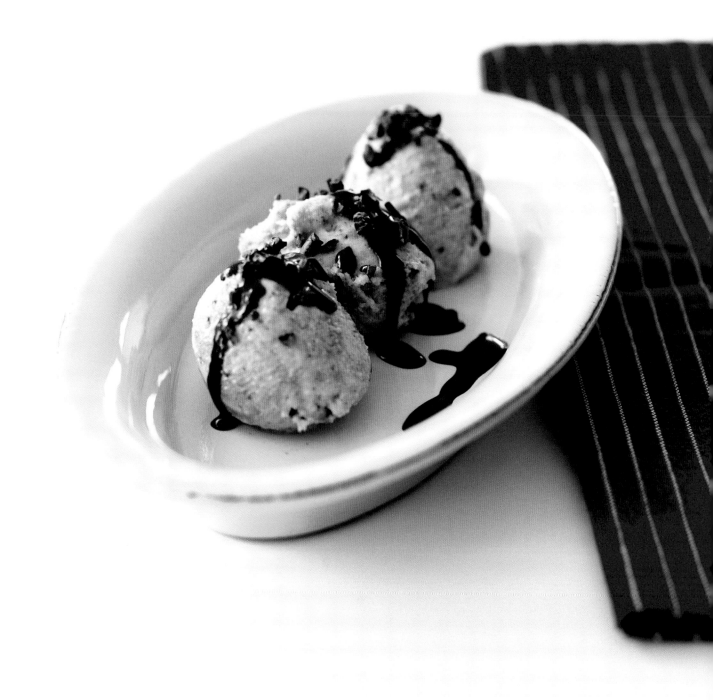

Chocolate Mousse

1 avocado
20 dates, pitted
3–4 tablespoons raw cacao
4 tablespoons agave nectar
Orange juice and some grated orange zest (optional)

Peel the avocado and remove the pit. Mix all the ingredients in a blender and blend until creamy.

Garnish with a slice of orange, kiwi, or fresh strawberries.

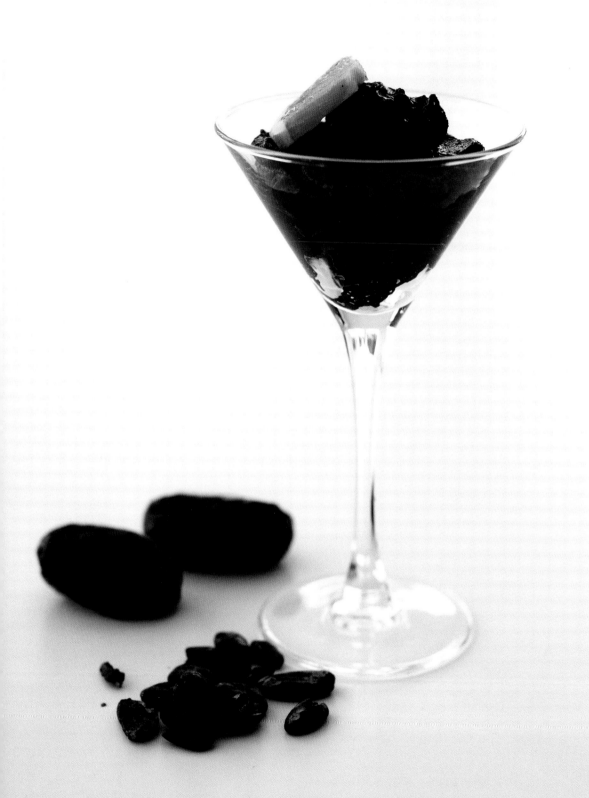

Crust:
1 cup (2½ dls) macadamia nuts or hazelnuts
5 dates, pitted
¼ cup (½ dl) coconut flour

Filling:
2½ cups (6 dls) cashews, soaked 2 hours
2 tablespoons lemon juice
¼ cup (½ dl) water
½ cup (1 dl) raw honey
½ cup (1 dl) coconut oil
1 teaspoon vanilla
¼ teaspoon salt

Garnish:
1 cup (250 g) strawberries
Chocolate sauce (p. 260)

Blend the macadamia nuts and dates in a food processor until you have a compact mass. Place wax paper, plastic wrap, or aluminum foil in a pie dish and sprinkle with coconut flour. Spread the mass of nuts and dates in the dish.

Mix all ingredients for the filling in a food processor until it becomes a smooth mass. Spread this mixture on top of the crust and place the dish in the refrigerator until the cake has set.

Cut the fresh strawberries into halves and arrange them on the cake. Serve with chocolate sauce.

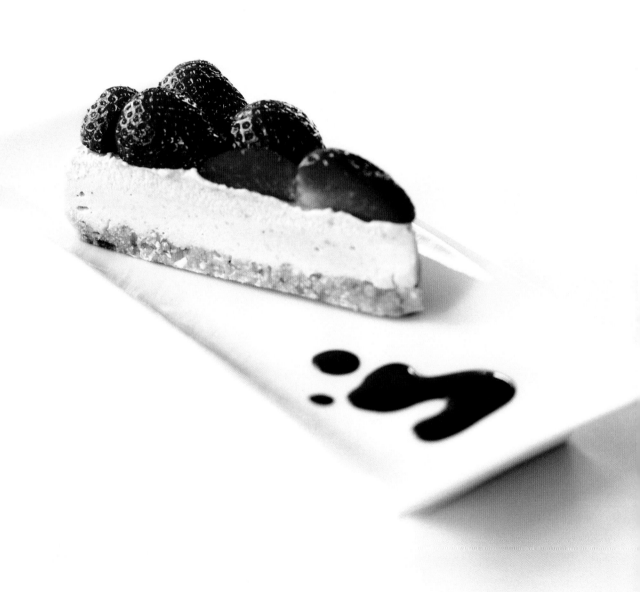

Kiwi Sorbet

1 cup (250 g) kiwifruit
¾ cup (200 g) dates, pitted
Vanilla, cardamom, or cinnamon (optional)

Peel the kiwis, cut them into small pieces, and freeze them in freezer bags.

Blend the dates and frozen kiwis in a food processor until you have a delicious, creamy sorbet.

You can substitute raspberries or other berries for the kiwis.

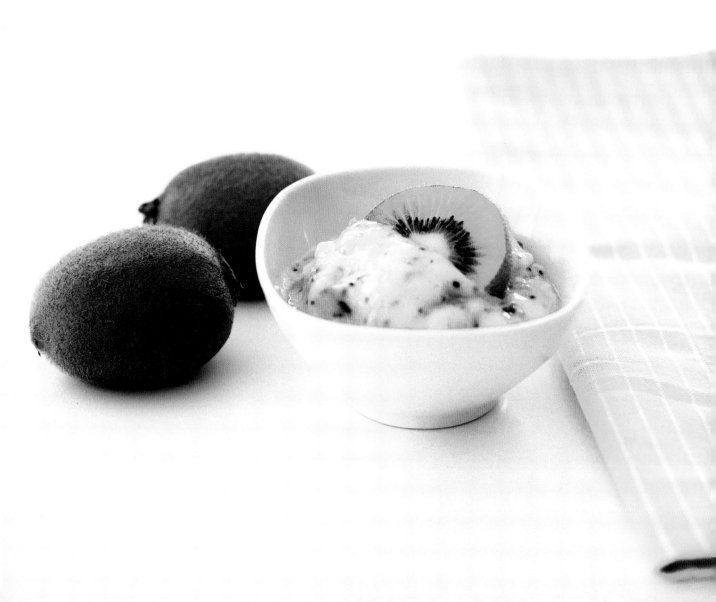

Raspberry-Orange Soup

10 oranges
1¼ cup (300 g) cashews
1 handful fresh mint
1 cup (250 g) raspberries

1 teaspoon cinnamon
2 tablespoons raw honey

Grate a little orange zest and save for garnishing, along with a few mint leaves. Juice the oranges and mix orange juice with nuts, mint, and raspberries in the blender. Blend until you have a nicely colored soup. Add cinnamon and honey to taste.

Garnish with orange zest and mint leaves.

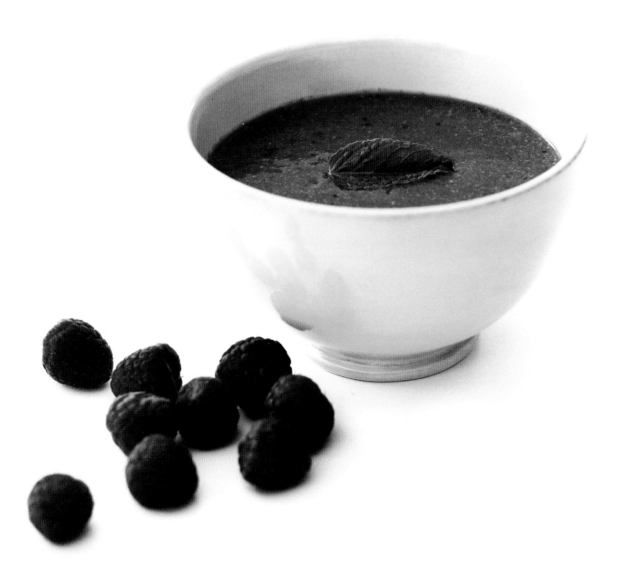

Super Simple Vanilla Ice Cream

4 ripe bananas
1 teaspoon vanilla
Raw cacao nibs (optional)

Peel the bananas, cut them into small pieces, and freeze them in freezer bags. Blend the frozen bananas in a food processor for 1 minute. Add vanilla and blend until the mixture looks like ice cream.

Serve immediately.

Always have frozen bananas in the freezer ready for ice cream and smoothies.

Banana Split

1 banana per person
3 scoops of your favorite ice cream
Heavenly vanilla cream (p. 262)
Chopped hazelnuts or almonds
Chocolate sauce (p. 260)

Arrange on a plate. Enjoy!

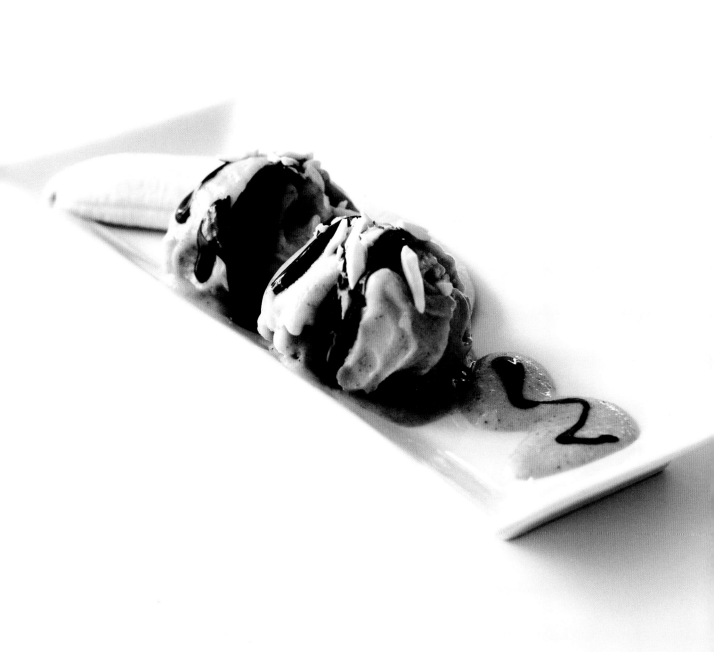

Strawberries Dipped in Chocolate

Strawberries
Chocolate sauce (p. 260)

Rinse the strawberries and make the chocolate sauce. Dip the strawberries in the chocolate and put them in the refrigerator, stems down, to set for an hour.

A classic—but now as raw food. Simple but fantastic!

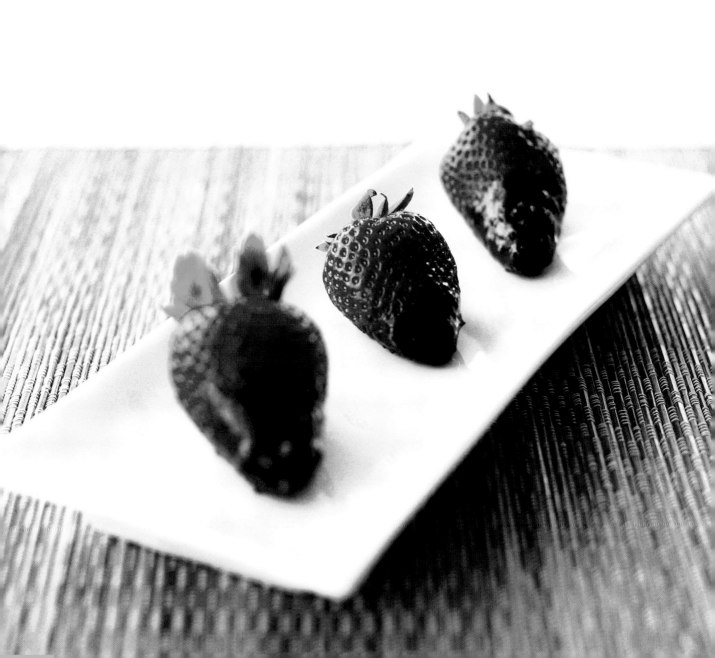

Pineapple Carpaccio with Berry Coulis

1 pineapple

¼ cup (½ dl) agave nectar
Berry coulis (p. 266)
Mint leaves

Cut the top and bottom off the pineapple and peel. Cut it lengthwise into as thin slices as possible. Layer the slices on plastic wrap, with wrap between each layer. Freeze the slices for 1–2 hours.

Arrange on a plate and top with agave, coulis, and mint leaves.

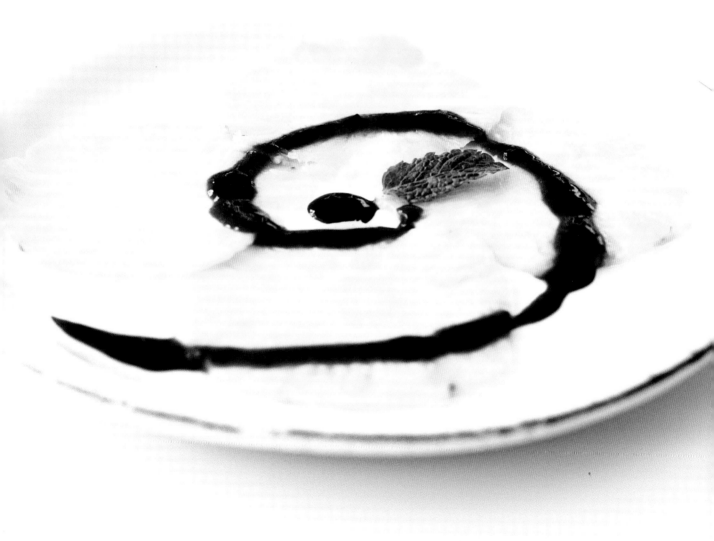

Strawberry Ice Cream

4 ripe bananas
½ cup (125 g) strawberries
3–4 tablespoons agave nectar
1 teaspoon vanilla

Strawberries can easily be replaced by mango, blackberries, black currant, or similar fruits.

Use the same procedure for this ice cream as for the super simple vanilla ice cream on page 222. You will have the most enchanting strawberry ice cream in less than 5 minutes. If it is too soft, put it in the freezer before serving.

Adjust the amount of agave nectar according to how sour the berries are.

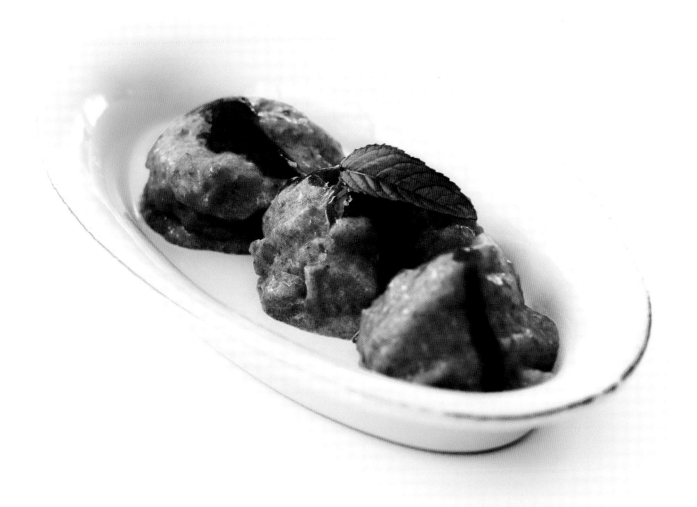

Delicious Mango-Raspberry Cocktail

2 mangoes
1 cup (250 g) raspberries

Garnish:
1 tablespoon agave nectar
Cacao nibs
Mint leaves

Peel and remove pits from the mangoes and blend the fruit meat. Blend the raspberries separately.

Arrange the two sorbets in a wineglass in alternating layers. Pour the agave nectar on top, sprinkle with cacao nibs, and finish off with a mint leaf or two.

Serve ice-cold to highlight the flavor from the sweet mangoes and the sour raspberries.

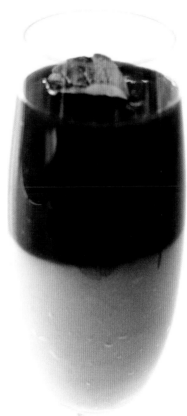

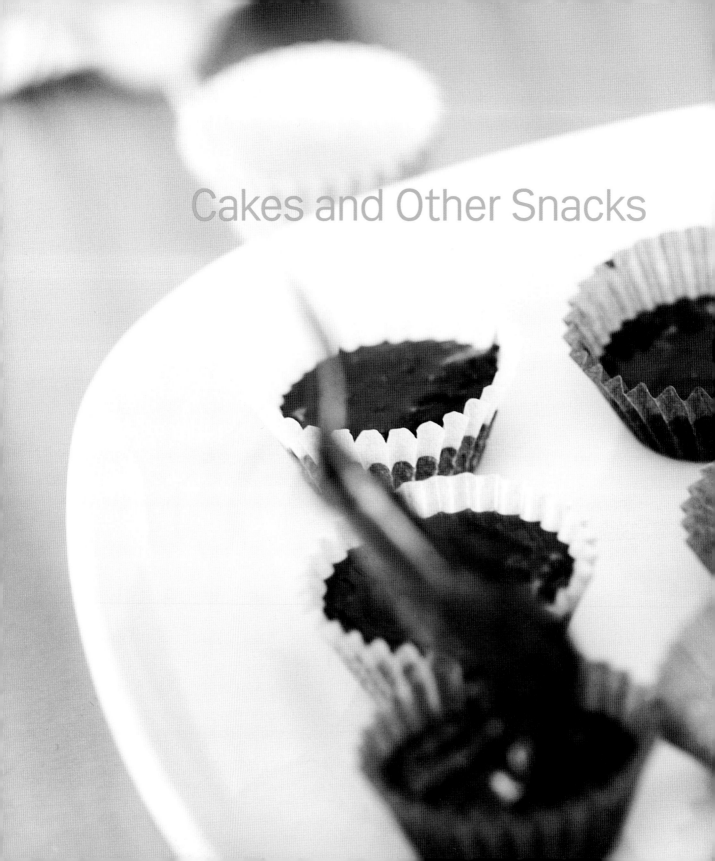

Cakes and Other Snacks

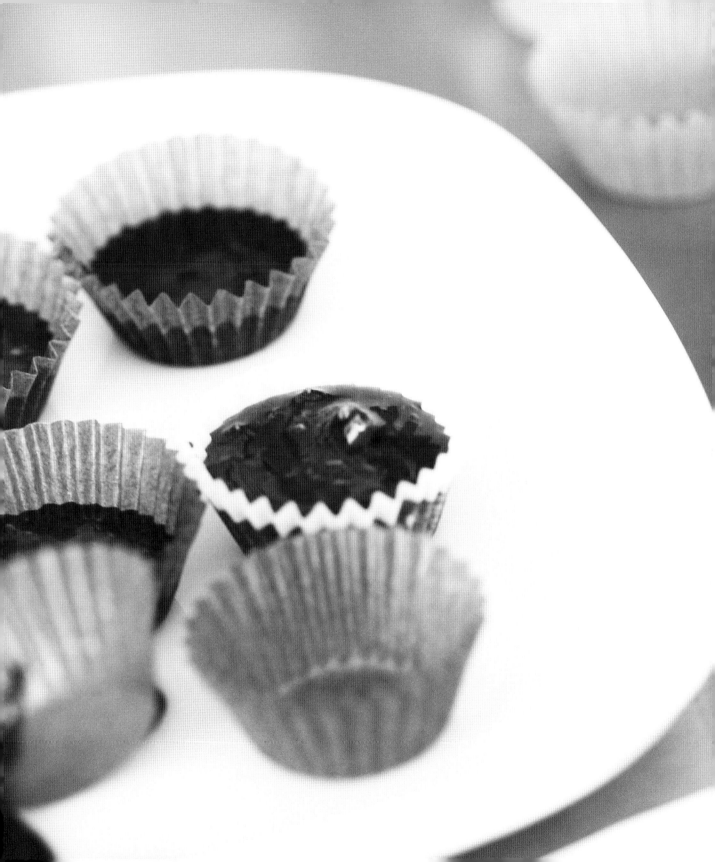

Carrot Cake

1¼ cups (3 dls) oatmeal
½ cup (1 dl) hazelnuts
¾ cup (2 dls) dates, soaked
8 carrots
1 teaspoon vanilla
1 teaspoon cinnamon
½ teaspoon cardamom
½ cup (1 dl) raisins

1 cup (2½ dls) cashews
Juice of ½ orange
4 tablespoons raw honey

Garnish:
Grated orange zest

Grind the oatmeal in a coffee grinder or with a hand blender. Do the same with the nuts. Remove pits from the dates and cut them into small pieces. Peel the carrots, cut them into small pieces, and blend well in a food processor. Add dates, flour (oatmeal and nuts), vanilla, cinnamon, and cardamom, and blend. Then add the raisins and blend.

Pour into a pie dish and leave it to stand in the refrigerator.

Chop the cashews very finely with a hand blender, add juice and honey, and stir until you have a delicious, thick cream.

Just before serving, pour the cream on top of the cake and garnish with orange zest.

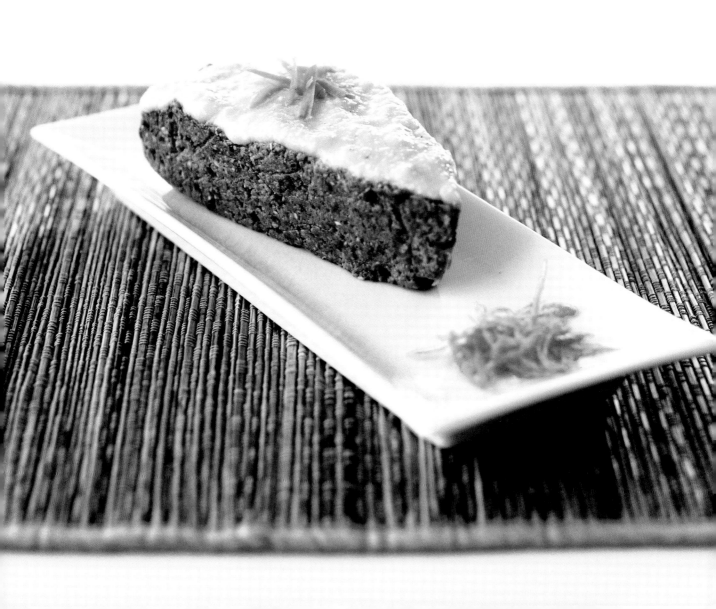

Easy Apple Cake

4 apples, cored
½ cup (1 dl) raisins
1 tablespoon cinnamon

¾ cup (1½ dls) hazelnuts
½ cup (1 dl) oatmeal

"You Just Might Think It's Crème Fraîche" (p. 262)
Apricot jam (p. 264) or finely chopped raisins

Blend apples, raisins, and cinnamon in a food processor. Chop the nuts and oatmeal in a blender or a coffee grinder.

Layer the mashed apple and chopped nuts in alternating layers. Finish off with a top layer of apricot jam or finely chopped raisins.

Serve with crème fraîche.

You can easily change this cake to an apple pie by adding the mashed apple mixture to a nut crust. Do not use oatmeal but chop the nuts finely and sprinkle on top of the mashed apples. Garnish with apple slices.

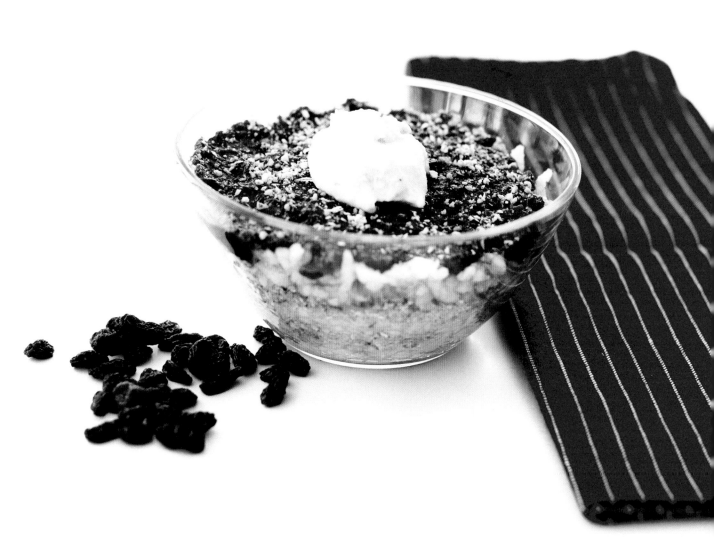

Marzipan

2 cups (5 dls) almonds
½ cup (1 dl) raw honey

Allow the almonds to soak overnight. Remove their skins and blend the nuts in a food processor until they turn to flour. Remember to stop the machine frequently in order to avoid overheating. Continue blending until the almonds start to become moist. Add the honey a little at a time.

You can serve the marzipan as it is or enjoy it with Quetzalcoatl chocolate (see page 256). You can also try making it into a roulade with a peach filling.

This marzipan is suitable to use the way you normally use marzipan.

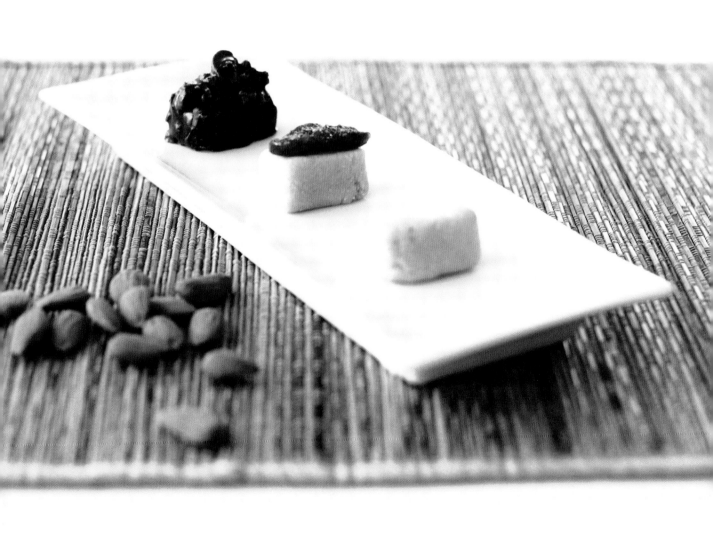

Banana and Cashews in Cinnamon

When I feel like a quick snack!

1 banana
1 handful cashews
½ teaspoon cinnamon

Peel a banana and cut it into thin slices. Rough-chop the nuts and mix them together with the banana and cinnamon.

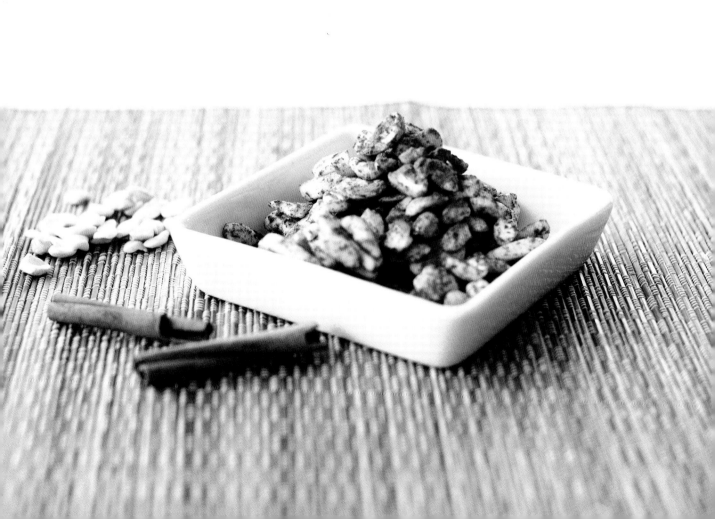

Lemon Pie

Crust:
2 cups (5 dls) dates
2 cups (5 dls) walnuts or mixed nuts

Filling:
1¾ cups (4 dls) dates
1 teaspoon vanilla
2 teaspoons raw cacao
Juice of 1 lemon
1 tablespoon coconut oil or chocolate butter

Garnish:
Grated lemon zest
Coconut flour

Blend the dates and walnuts in a food processor until they form a moist mass. This is the dough for the crust. Spread the mass on wax paper or aluminum foil in a pie dish.

For the filling, blend the dates, vanilla, cacao, lemon juice, and the coconut oil or chocolate butter in a food processor until creamy. Place the filling in the crust and leave the pie in the refrigerator for at least 3 hours. Garnish with grated lemon zest and coconut flour and serve.

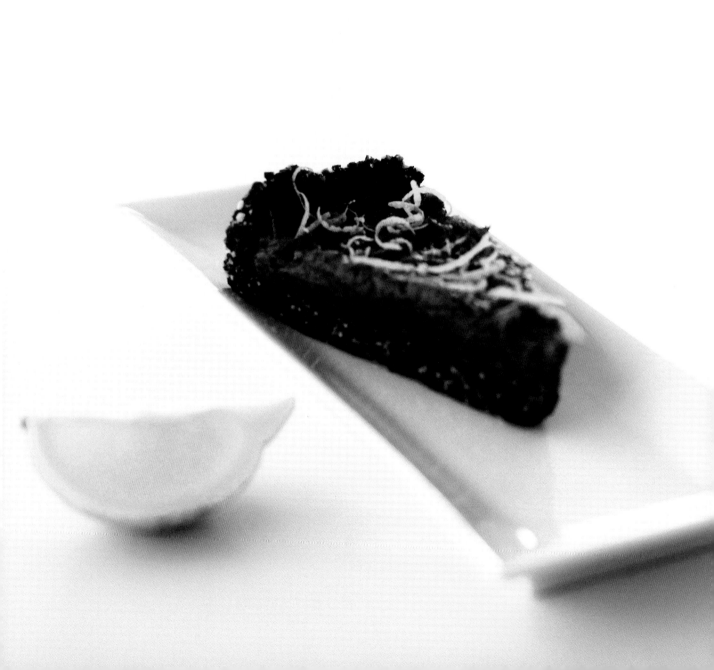

Raspberry Tart with Nut Crust

Crust:
2 cups (5 dls) raisins
2 cups (5 dls) hazelnuts

Filling:
1¾ cups (4 dls) dates
Juice of ½ lime

Garnish:
1¼ cups (300 g) raspberries

Blend the raisins and nuts in a food processor until they form a moist mass. This is the dough for the crust. Spread the mass on wax paper in a pie dish.

If the dates are very dry, soak them before use. Blend the dates and lime juice in a food processor until creamy. Place the filling in the crust and leave the pie in the refrigerator for at least 3 hours. Garnish with raspberries and serve.

You can vary this pie with all kinds of fillings.

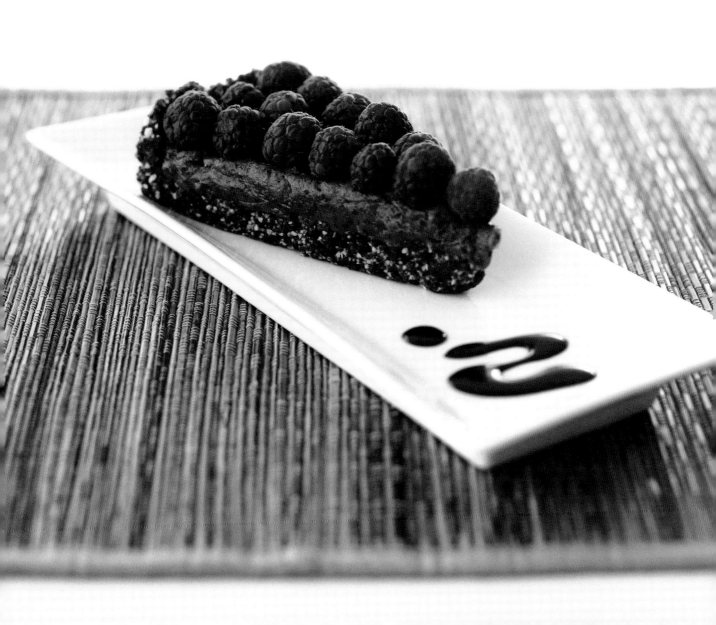

Coconut Puffs

1¼ cups (3 dls) macadamia nuts, soaked for 3–4 hours
2 cups (5 dls) coconut flour
¼ cup (½ dl) agave nectar
3 tablespoons coconut oil
1 teaspoon vanilla

Using a hand blender, chop the nuts until they are like rough flour.

Mix all the ingredients together in a bowl using a good wooden spoon until you have a solid mass. Use your fingers to form tiny coconut puffs and place them on a plate lined with wax paper. When all the puffs are made, cover them with aluminum foil and let them set in the refrigerator. After a couple of hours they are ready to serve. If you like, drizzle the puffs with chocolate sauce (p. 260).

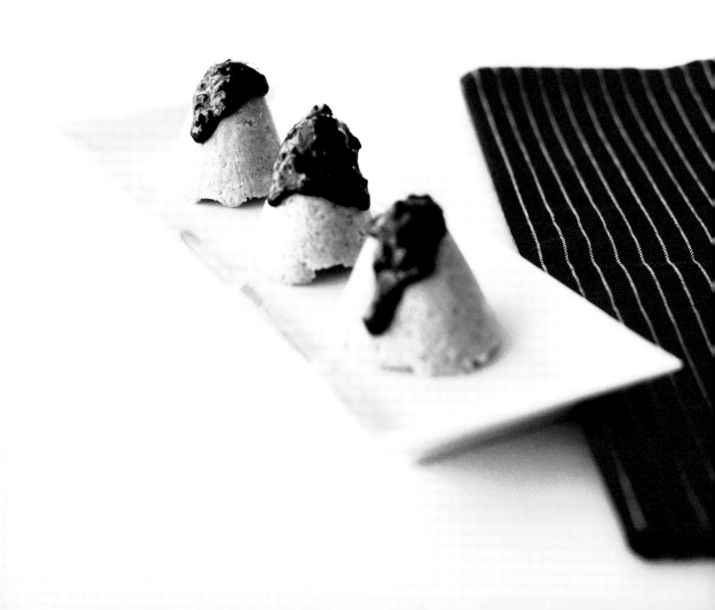

Crust:
¾ cup (2 dls) nuts
½ cup (1 dl) raw cacao
1½ tablespoons coconut oil
1 pinch of salt

Filling:
¾ cup (2 dls) raw cacao
2½ cups (600 g) dates
3 tablespoons coconut oil
2 teaspoons vanilla
½ teaspoon salt

Garnish:
Fresh raspberries

Grind nuts into flour in a coffee grinder. Stir cacao, coconut oil, and salt with the nut flour until you get a solid mass. You can also use a food processor.

Spread the mass in as thin a layer as possible in a pie dish lined with wax paper.

Mix the ingredients for the filling in a food processor until creamy. Pour the filling into the pie dish and leave it in the refrigerator for a couple of hours. If it has to be served quickly, you can place it in the freezer for about an hour instead.

Serve on a plate with fresh raspberries or try with passion fruit.

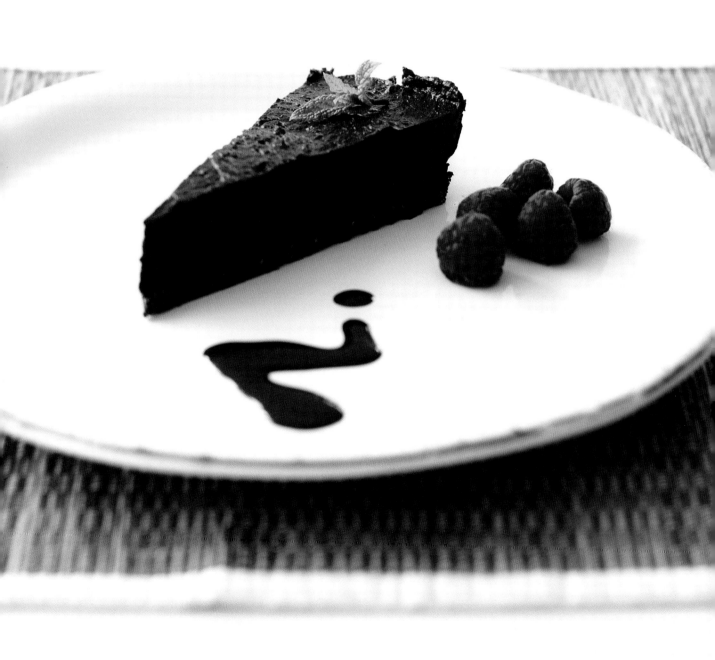

Crust:
1¾ cups (4 dls) pecan nuts
½ cup (1 dl) coconut flour
1¼ cups (3 dls) dates

Filling:
2 cups (500 g) strawberries
1–2 ripe bananas
1 teaspoon vanilla
½ cup (100 g) cashews
1 tablespoon psyllium husks or crushed linseed
Agave nectar (optional)

Blend nuts in a food processor until they are finely ground. Add coconut flour and dates. Soak dates before use if they are too dry.

Cover a pie dish with wax paper and spread the mass inside the entire dish so that it also covers the edges.

Mix half of the strawberries and banana with the vanilla in a food processor. Blend until creamy. Add extra vanilla and agave nectar to taste.

Pour the cream into the pie dish. Cut the rest of the strawberries into halves and arrange them on top. Leave the pie in the refrigerator for an hour, then serve.

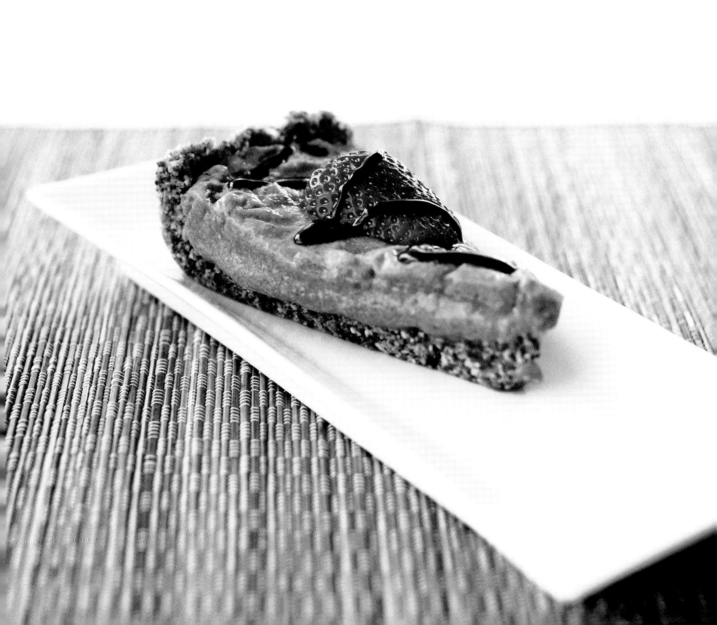

Confectionary Rolls

1 cup (2½ dls) cashews
1¼ cups (300 g) dates
1 cup (2½ dls) coconut flour
¼ cup (½ dl) orange juice or water
2–4 tablespoons raw cacao
1 teaspoon vanilla
1 pinch of cayenne pepper
Grated orange zest (optional)

Coconut flour for decorating the rolls

Chop the nuts finely in a food processor. Add the rest of the ingredients and blend until it is solid and starts to become lumpy. Add extra cacao if necessary, and add water if the dough is too dry.

Take a good handful of the dough and roll it into a log shape approximately 1 inch (3 cm) thick. Roll the log in the coconut flour. You can also shape small balls and roll them in the coconut flour.

Leave in the refrigerator or freezer overnight.

Try different flavors in your rolls using ingredients such as carob, lime, mint, or cloves.

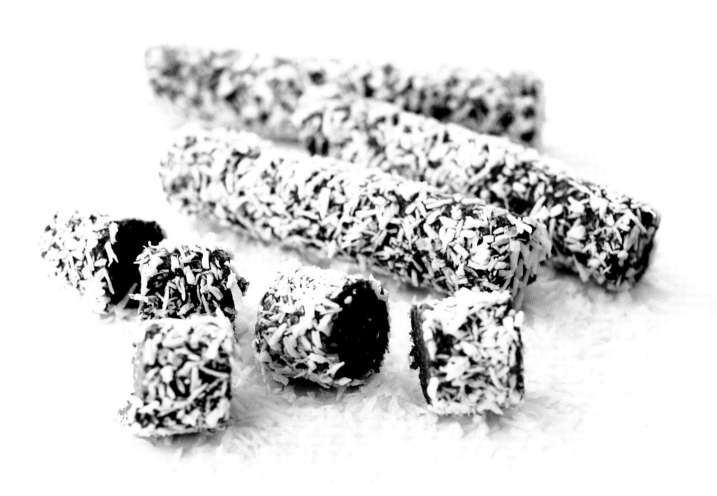

Blueberry Tart

Crust:
1¼ cups (3 dls) nuts
¾ cup (2 dls) dried apricots

Filling:
2½ cups (6 dls) blueberries
1¾ cups (4 dls) cashews or macadamia nuts
½ cup (1 dl) agave nectar
1–2 tablespoons raw cacao

If the apricots aren't soft, soak them in water for a couple of hours. Blend the nuts in a blender or coffee grinder until they are finely ground. Mix the apricots and ground nuts in a food processor until the mixture forms a ball shape.

Cover a pie dish with wax paper and spread the dough throughout the dish so that it covers the edges as well. Leave the dough in the refrigerator.

Blend most of the blueberries, saving a handful for garnish. Add cashews, agave nectar, and cacao and blend until creamy.

Pour the blueberry filling into the tin and garnish with blueberries. Leave the tart in the refrigerator for a couple of hours before serving.

This tart is wonderful and has the most beautiful colors.

You could also replace half the nuts in the base with oatmeal.

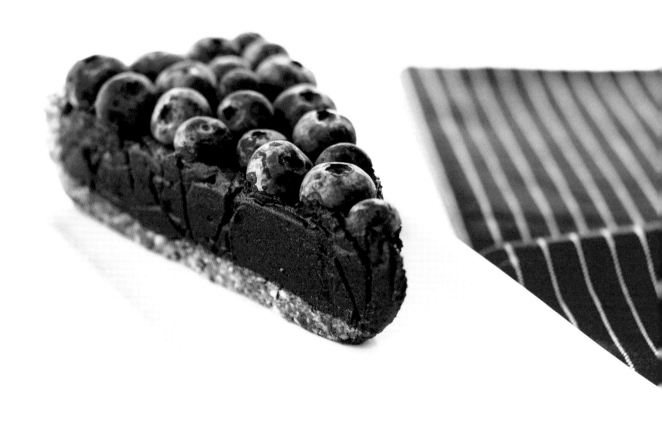

Quetzalcoatl Chocolate

According to an ancient Mesoamerican myth, Quetzalcoatl is the God of Snakes who brought the cacao bean from heaven to Earth.

½ cup (1 dl) goji berries
Juice of 1 orange
½ cup (1 dl) cashews
5 tablespoons raw cacao
½ cup (1 dl) agave nectar
1 tablespoon coconut oil
1 pinch of cayenne pepper

Let the berries soak in orange juice for at least an hour, then drain them. Save the juice for some other use or drink it. Chop the nuts finely in a coffee grinder.

Stir the cacao into the agave nectar little by little to make chocolate. Add the rest of the ingredients and stir.

Pour the chocolate into mini muffin molds and leave in the refrigerator for a couple of hours.

If you want pure dark chocolate, without any gojis or cayenne, mix together just the agave nectar, raw cacao, and coconut oil.

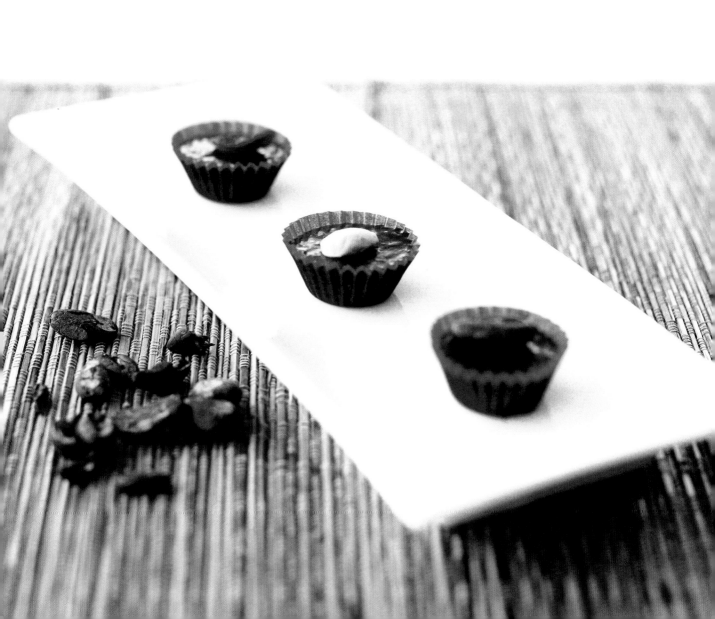

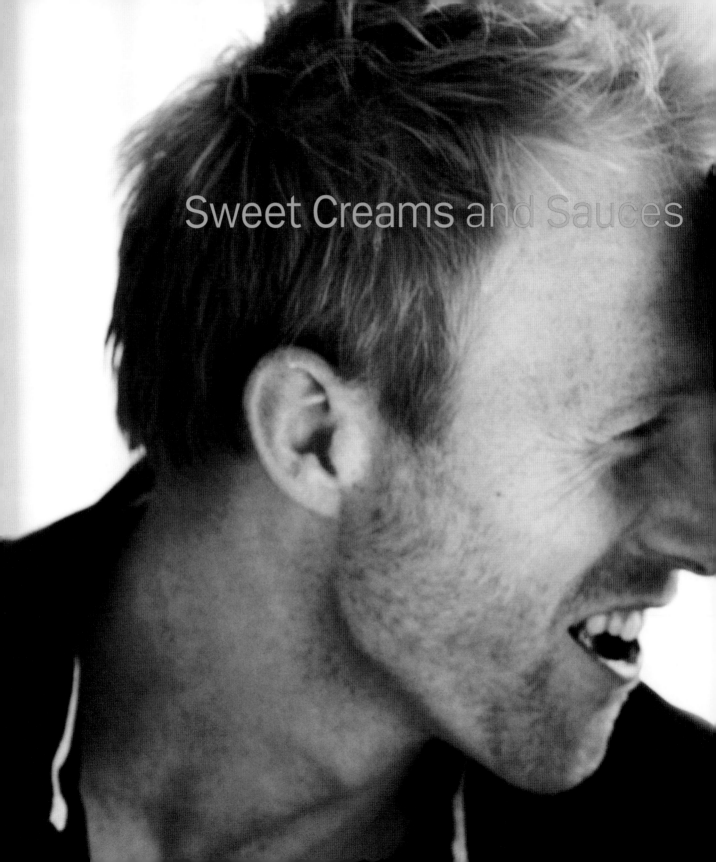

Sweet Creams and Sauces

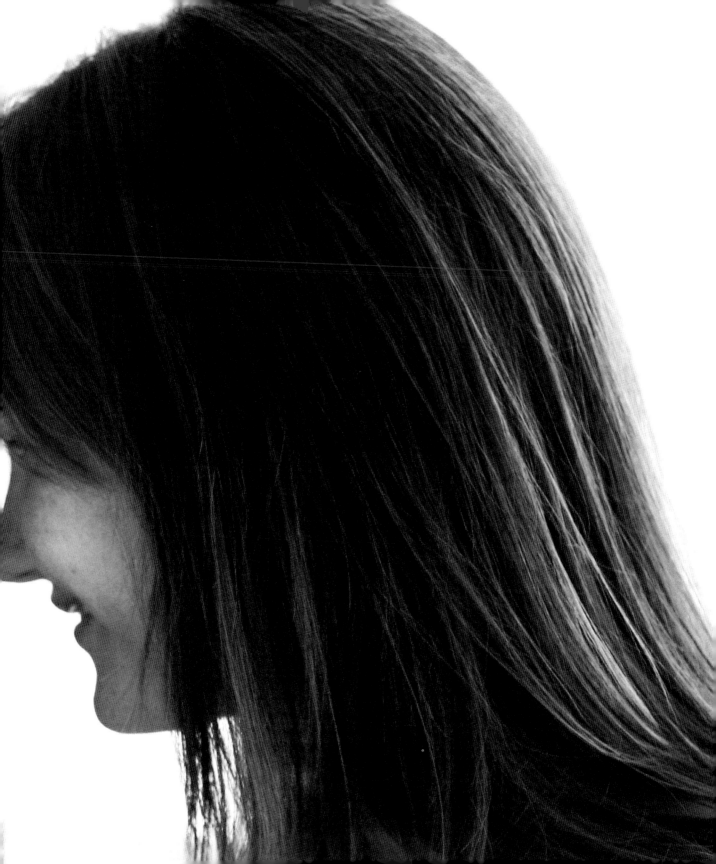

Coconut Cream

1 coconut (all of the milk, ¼ of the meat)
½ cup (1 dl) agave nectar
1 teaspoon vanilla
Water as needed

Mix all the ingredients in a food processor with water until it reaches the desired consistency.

Chocolate Sauce

½ cup (1 dl) neutral-tasting oil
½ cup (1 dl) cacao
⅓ cup (¾ dl) agave nectar

Mix the three ingredients together in a small jar or dish.

This sauce is wonderful with ice cream. I often use it for decorating plates when I serve desserts and cakes.

Replace oil with ⅓ cup (¾ dls) water or nut milk if you find the sauce too oily.

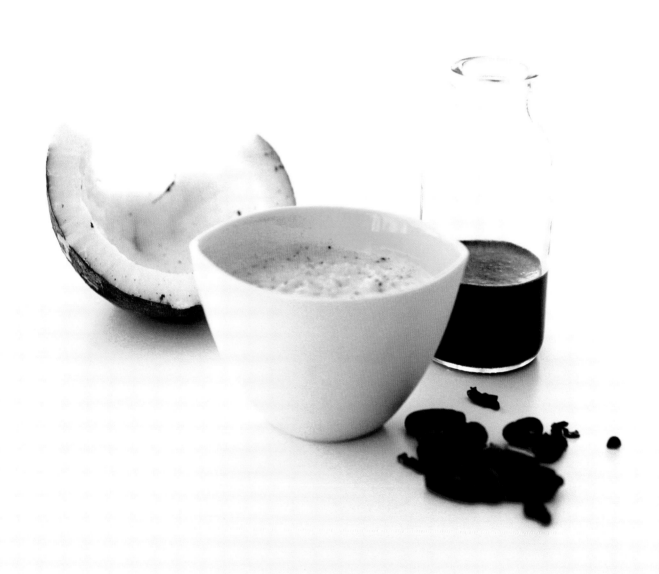

"You Just Might Think It's Crème Fraîche"

1 cup (2½ dls) cashews, soaked for 2 hours
⅓ cup (¾ dl) water
1–2 teaspoons apple cider vinegar or lemon juice
¼ teaspoon salt

Drain the nuts and mix all the ingredients together with a hand blender.

The cream will thicken if you leave it for a while because the nuts absorb the water.

Heavenly Vanilla Cream

¾ cup (2 dls) cashews
½ cup (1 dl) water
3 tablespoons agave nectar
2 teaspoons vanilla

Mix all the ingredients in a tall bowl with a hand blender, adding the water slowly.

The cream will thicken if you leave it for a while because the nuts absorb the water.

You can use orange juice instead of water or substitute other nuts for the cashews.

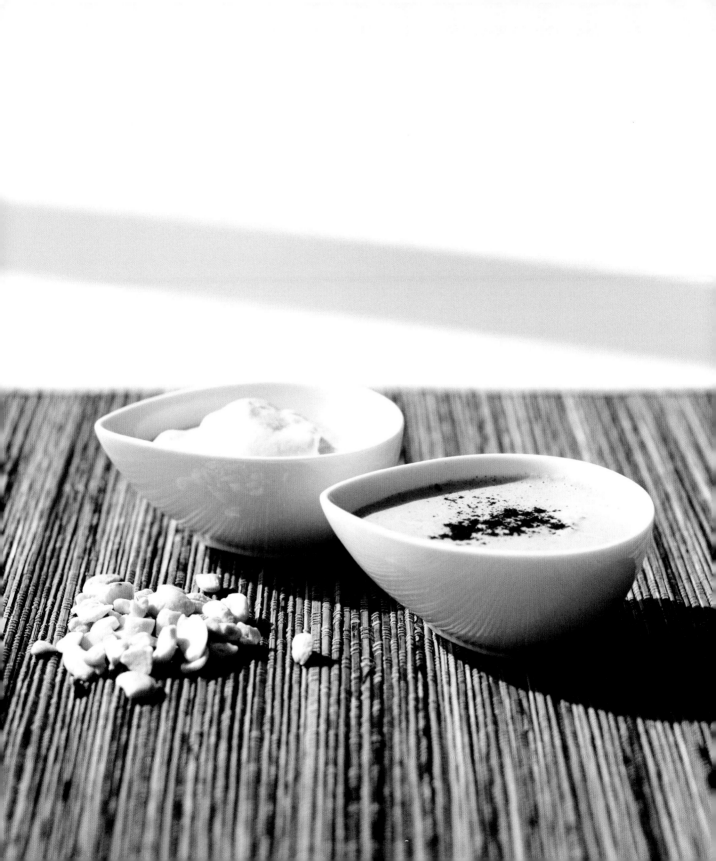

Apricot Jam

¾ cup (2 dls) dried apricots
Juice of 1 orange
½ cup (1 dl) strawberries
1 teaspoon cinnamon

Soak the apricots in the orange juice, remove the strawberry stems, and mix all the ingredients together in a blender.

Make your own jam: fast, easy, and tasty.

In autumn, when the plum trees are full of ripe plums, you can use them instead of apricots.

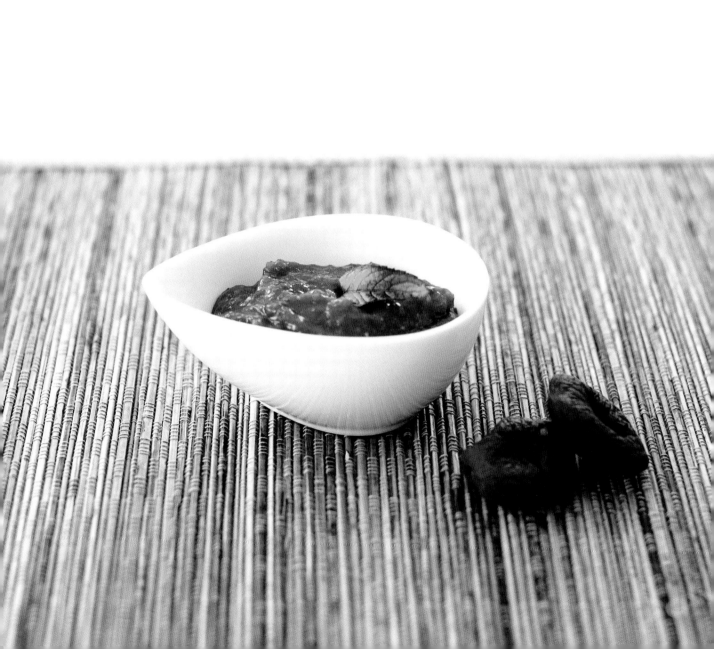

Date Syrup

1¼ cups (3 dls) dates, pitted
1¼ cups (3 dls) water

Blend the ingredients. Pour the syrup into a bottle and leave it in the refrigerator. This syrup can be used as a sweetener instead of honey or agave.

Berry Coulis

1 cup (250 g) berries
1–4 tablespoons agave nectar

Mix berries and agave in a blender. If needed, add extra agave to taste.

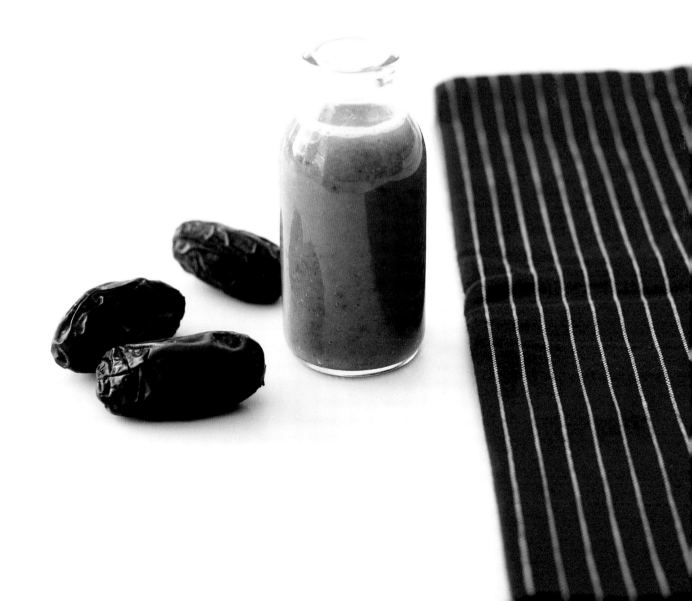

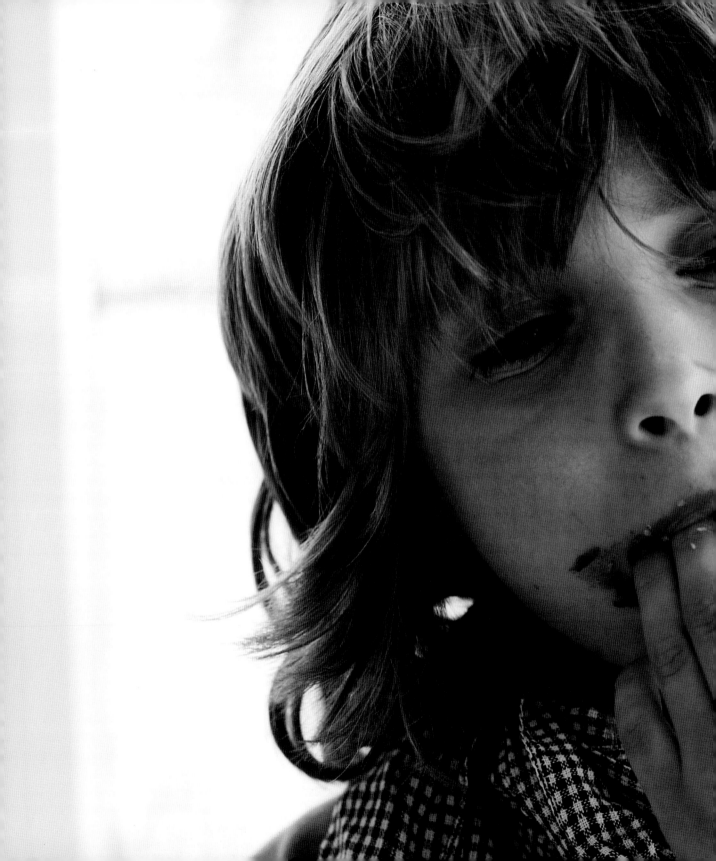

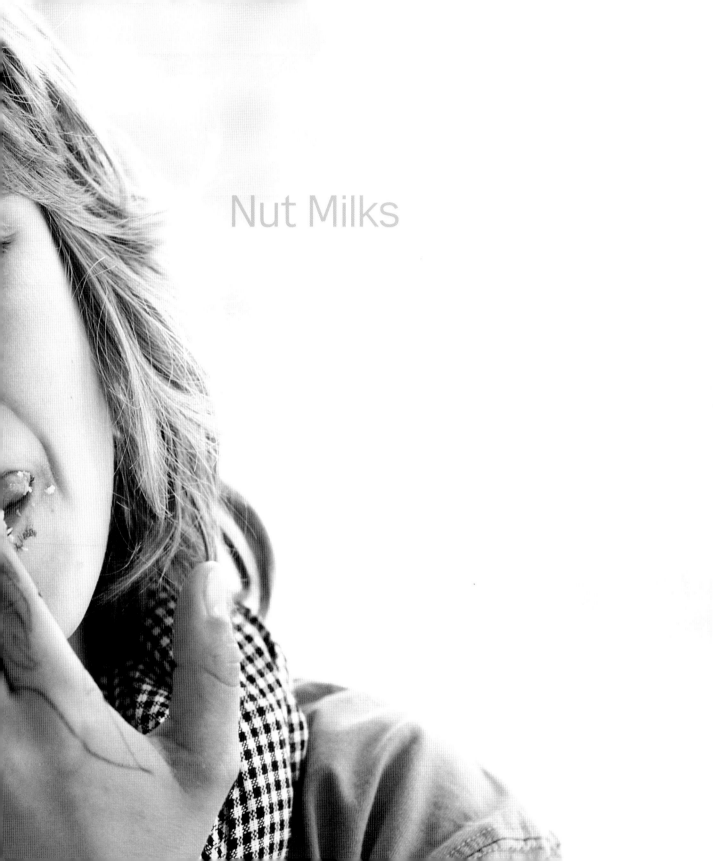

Nut Milks

Almond Milk

¾ cup (2 dls) almonds
2½–3½ cups (6–8 dls) water
3 tablespoons raw honey
1 pinch of salt (optional)

Let the almonds soak for 10–12 hours. Drain almonds. Mix all the ingredients in a blender until you have the most delicious almond milk.

If you like, you can strain the milk using a fine-meshed sieve or a nut milk bag. The leftovers can be used as nut crumbles for tarts or pies.

For those of you who didn't have the time to soak the almonds, don't worry—you can still make the milk. The advantage of soaking the almonds is that they become easier to digest and the nutrients are easier to absorb. It also becomes possible to remove the skins, which makes the milk even more delicious.

Chocolate Milk

2½ cups (6 dls) of your favorite nut milk
2 tablespoons raw cacao or carob powder
¼ cup (½ dl) orange juice
1 tablespoon coconut oil
Cinnamon, vanilla, and/or cardamom (optional)

Mix all ingredients and serve. Yummy!

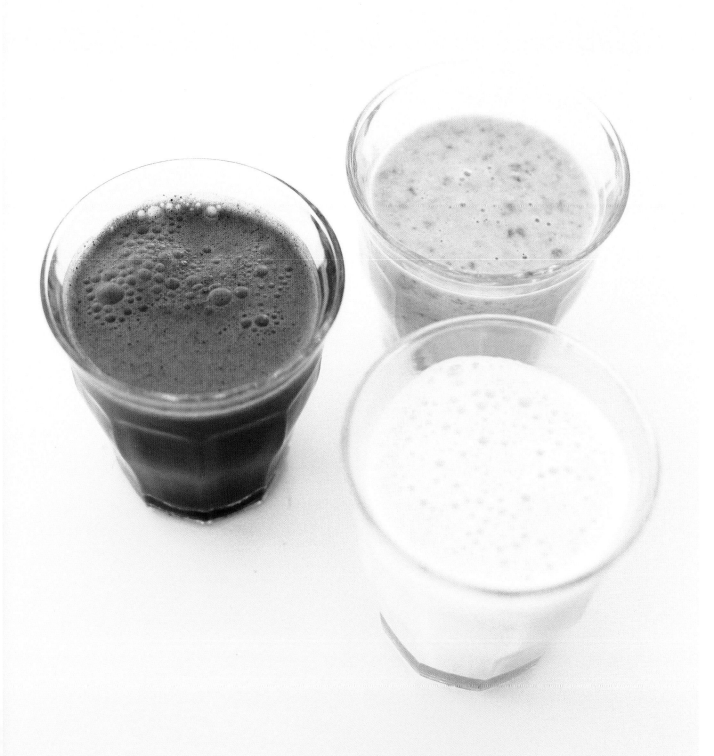

Cashew Nut Milk

¾ cup (2 dls) cashews
2½–3½ cups (6–8 dls) water
3 tablespoons agave nectar
1 pinch of cardamom or vanilla powder
Salt (optional)

Use the same procedure as in the recipe for almond milk, above. Cashews have to soak for only a couple of hours, unlike almonds, which need to soak for 10–12 hours.

You can add more salt or sweetener depending on whether the milk is used for a main dish (entrée) or for a dessert.

Rooibos Nut Milk

¾ cup (2 dls) nuts
2½–3½ cups (6–8 dls) cold rooibos tea
3 tablespoons agave nectar

Use the same procedure as for almond milk, but make the rooibos tea first and let it cool.

Good for breakfast, for smoothies, or just as a refreshing drink on its own.

Also try with green tea, green strawberry tea, or your own favorite tea.

Strawberry Milk

¾ cup (2 dls) nuts
2½–3½ cups (6–8 dls) water
4–5 tablespoons agave nectar
1 handful fresh strawberries, destemmed
½ teaspoon vanilla

Mix all the ingredients in a blender. Add frozen strawberries on a hot summer day or leave the drink in the refrigerator for an hour to chill before serving.

Sesame or Sunflower Milk

¾ cup (2 dls) sesame seeds or sunflower seeds
1¾–2½ cups (4–6 dls) water
1 tablespoon agave nectar
Salt (optional)

Rinse the seeds and blend all the ingredients together in a blender.

Also good for use in more savory recipes since both of these seeds have a stronger and not-so-sweet taste.

Rice Milk

2 cups (5 dls) water
2–3 tablespoons rice bran powder
1 teaspoon agave nectar
½ teaspoon vanilla
1 pinch of salt

Mix all the ingredients in a blender and you get rice milk!

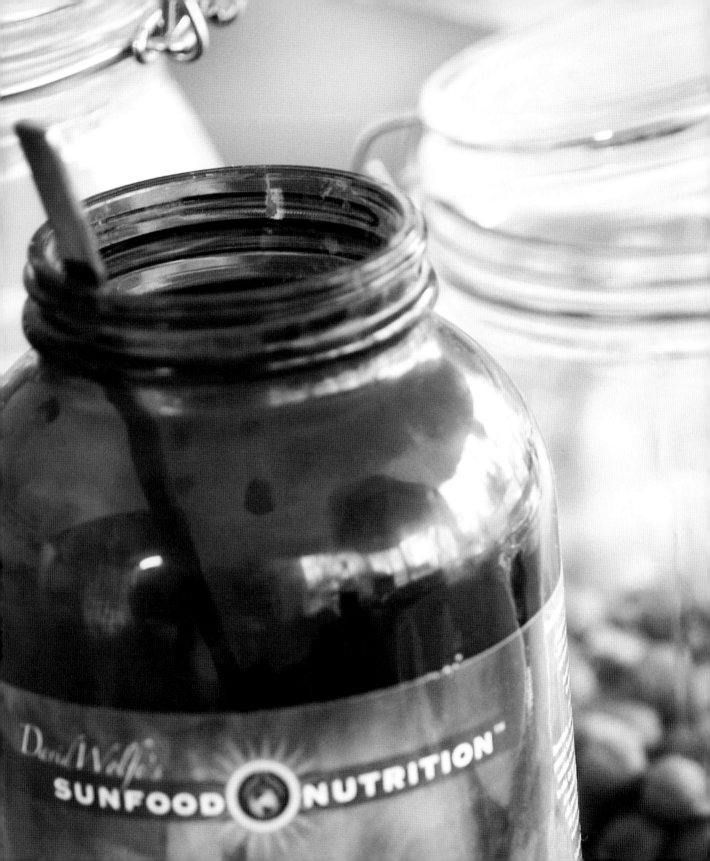

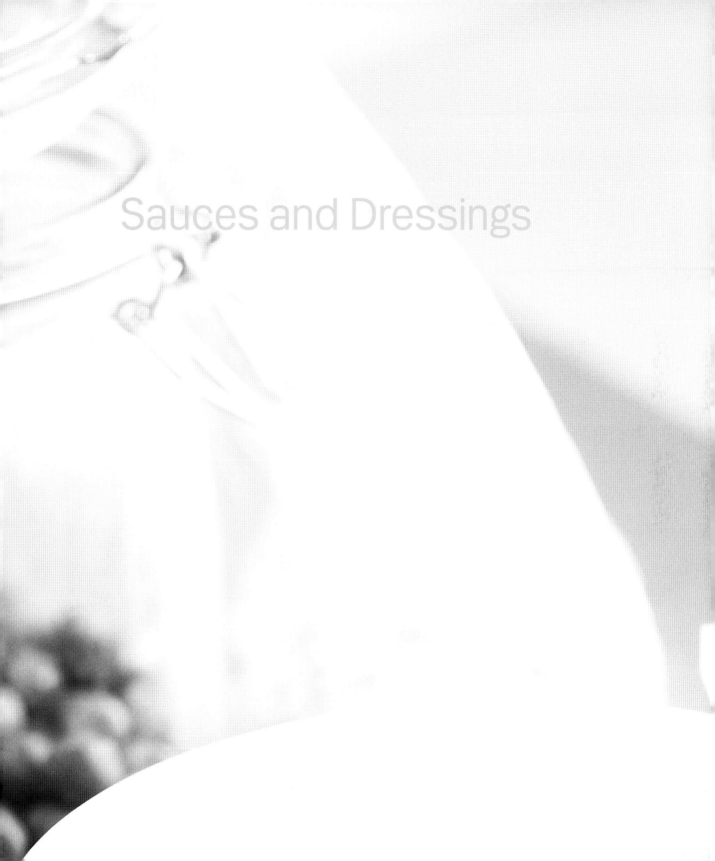

Sauces and Dressings

Sunflower and Beetroot Sauce

¾ cup (2 dls) sunflower seeds, soaked overnight
1 beetroot
2 teaspoons agave nectar
1 teaspoon lemon juice
½ teaspoon minced ginger
1 clove garlic, minced
Salt and pepper
Water

Grind the seeds in a mini grinder. Peel and dice the beetroot. Mix all the ingredients in a blender until you have a lovely colored creamy sauce.

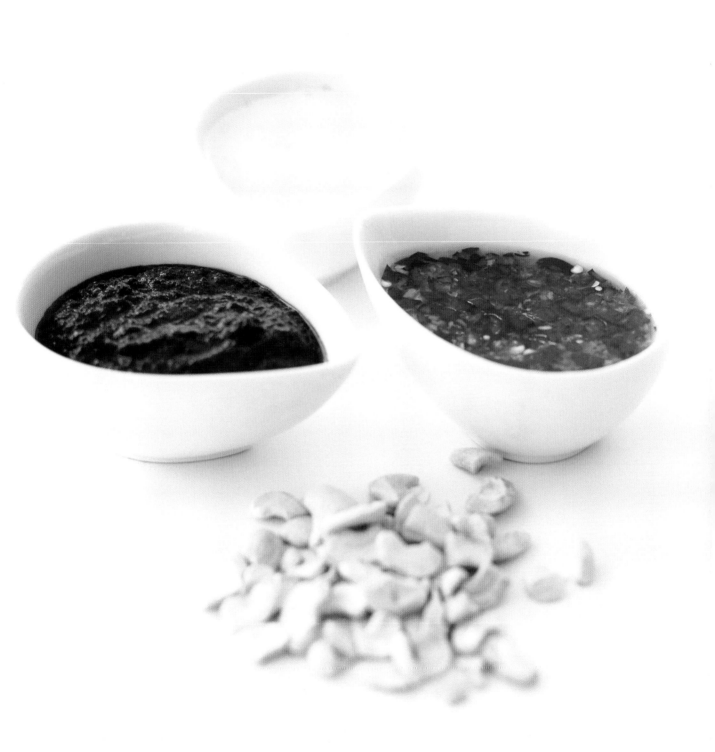

Pad Thai Sauce

¾ cup (1½ dls) cashew butter (p. 182)
½ cup (1 dl) water
1 tablespoon agave nectar
2 tablespoons lime juice
1 tablespoon Bragg Liquid Aminos, Nama Shoyu, or soy sauce
1 tablespoon minced ginger
1 tablespoon minced garlic
Chili pepper to taste
Salt and pepper

Mix all the ingredients in a blender. Add more water if necessary.

Super "Fish" Sauce

3–4 tablespoons seaweed
½ cup (1 dl) water
2 tablespoons dulse flakes
1 date, pitted
1 teaspoon Bragg Liquid Aminos, Nama Shoyu, or soy sauce
¼ teaspoon apple cider vinegar

Soak the seaweed until it's soft and blend with the rest of the ingredients in a blender.

Asian Sweet Chili Sauce

½ cup (1 dl) agave nectar
1–2 tablespoons apple cider vinegar
1 chili pepper
½–¾ inch (1–2 cm) ginger, minced

Stir the agave nectar and apple cider vinegar together. Finely chop the chili pepper and combine it and the minced ginger with the agave and vinegar mix. Stir a little and let it stand for a few hours to get the best benefit from the ginger and chili pepper.

Béchamel Sauce

½ cup (100 g) cashews
¾ cup (2 dls) avocado oil
½ cup (1 dl) water
Salt and pepper
1 teaspoon grated nutmeg

Mix cashews and oil with a hand blender. Add salt, pepper, and grated nutmeg to taste. Add water if necessary.

Basic Tomato Sauce

4 tomatoes
6 sun-dried tomatoes
½ red onion, chopped
3 tablespoons olive oil
2 cloves minced garlic
2 dates
1 teaspoon apple cider vinegar

Rosemary
Basil
Thyme
Salt and pepper

Soak the sun-dried tomatoes first if necessary.

Cut the tomatoes into quarters. Remove seeds and the wet tomato meat. Add all other ingredients to the rest of the tomatoes and blend.

Add herbs, salt, and pepper to taste.

Dressings

For many years I did not use dressings, but that was before I learned how to make my own. Even though I often eat salad without dressing, I have discovered that dressings are a good way of getting one's necessary daily amount of oil.

I prefer simple dressings and love experimenting.

You can easily make a large amount of dressing and keep it in the refrigerator for a couple of days, depending on the ingredients.

There are many ways of mixing a dressing. You can shake it, whisk it, stir with a fork, or use a hand blender or countertop blender. Sometimes all you need to do is toss the dressing ingredients in with the salad.

My Favorite Dressing with Honey and Dijon Mustard

½ cup (1 dl) olive oil
1 tablespoon raw honey
1 teaspoon Dijon mustard
¼ cup (⅓ dl) cider vinegar
1 pinch of salt

Stir or whisk the ingredients. Add more honey if you want it to be sweeter.

Fennel and Orange Dressing

Juice of 2 oranges
½ fennel bulb

Blend the orange juice and fennel together in a blender. A dressing without oil!

Easy Sour Dressing

½ cup (1 dl) olive oil
¼–½ cup (½–1 dl) apple cider vinegar
Salt and pepper to taste

Whisk or shake the ingredients until the oil and vinegar has mixed to a smooth dressing. You can control the sourness with the amount of vinegar you use.

Apple cider vinegar is fantastic for softening food. It helps your stomach acid do its job so you can draw maximum nourishment from your food.

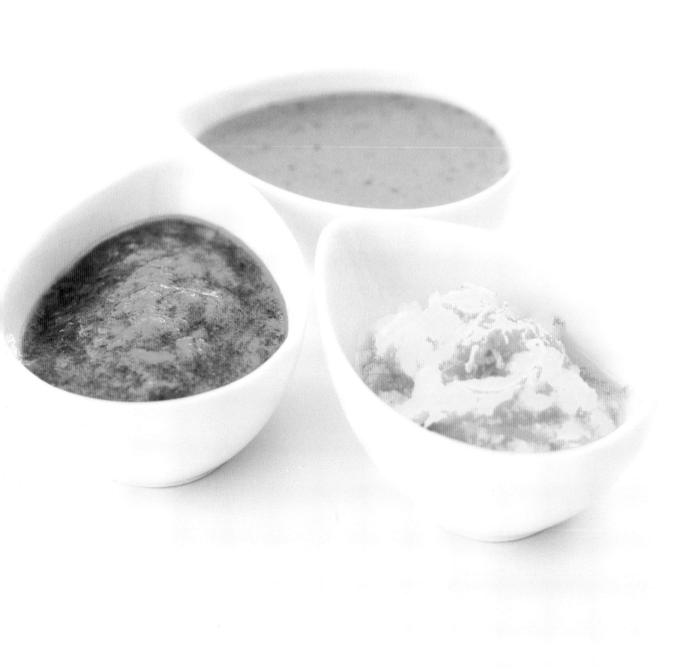

Scallion Dressing

2 scallions, chopped
¾ cup (2 dls) olive oil
⅓ cup (¾ dl) apple cider vinegar
¼ cup (½ dl) agave nectar
Salt and pepper

Blend all ingredients and add salt and pepper to taste.

Garlic Dressing

½ cup (1 dl) olive oil
1–2 cloves garlic
1 tablespoon chopped chives or parsley
1 tablespoon lemon juice
1 tablespoon tahini
Freshly ground salt and pepper

Stir, whisk, or blend all ingredients. If you use a blender, you do not have to chop the garlic.

If you don't like tahini, you can use sesame oil instead to achieve something of the same flavor.

Ginger and Soy Dressing

⅓ cup (¾ dl) sesame oil
¼ cup (½ dl) lemon juice
3 tablespoons agave nectar
2 tablespoons minced ginger
1 tablespoon Bragg Liquid Aminos, Nama Shoyu, or soy sauce

Blend, shake, or whisk all the ingredients together.

Horseradish Cream

¾ cup (200 g) cashews
¾ cup (2 dls) water
2 tablespoons olive oil
2 tablespoons agave nectar
2–4 tablespoons (30–50 g) grated horseradish
1 tablespoon minced onion
Salt and pepper

Blend all the ingredients together in a blender and add salt, pepper, and more horseradish to taste.

You can add more water or oil to make the most wonderful horseradish dressing.

Herbal Dressing

½ cup (1 dl) olive oil
1 handful fresh herbs (I mostly use parsley or basil)

This is the easiest dressing I know of. Just mix the ingredients in the salad.

Strawberry Vinaigrette

½ cup (1 dl) olive oil
¼ cup (½ dl) apple cider vinegar
¼ cup (½ dl) water
3–4 fresh strawberries, destemmed
1 teaspoon raw honey

Blend all the ingredients in a blender and add salt and pepper to taste.

Try experimenting with other berries.

Light Summer Dressing

1 cucumber, chopped
1 handful dill
½ handful mint leaves
1 tablespoon lemon juice or lime juice
Coarse Himalayan salt
Freshly ground pepper
Cumin (optional)

Set aside a few mint leaves and some dill for garnish. Mix all the other ingredients in a blender and add salt and pepper to taste.

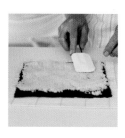

How to Roll Your Sushi Rolls

Spread cauliflower mix on top of a nori sheet, leaving about an inch (2–3 cm) at one end.

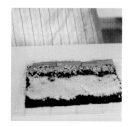

Start rolling from the end containing the filling.

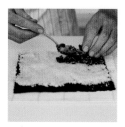

Form a line of red cabbage pâté on the cauliflower, towards the front edge of the nori sheet.

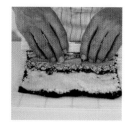

Carefully roll using a bamboo roller.

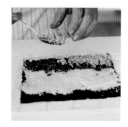

Add the pea pâté on top of the red cabbage pâté.

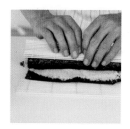

Stop when you get to the free end. Spread a little water on the seaweed end and roll the end.

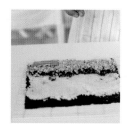

Put cashew butter on the carrot sticks and place them on top in a row.

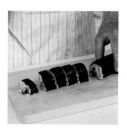

Use a very sharp knife to carefully cut the roll into sushi pieces.

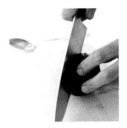

How to Dice an Avocado

How to cut an avocado without getting messy: Cut the avocado in half.

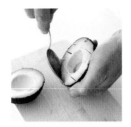

Remove the avocado mass with a spoon.

It's that easy!

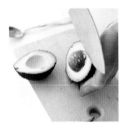

Remove the pit.

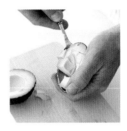

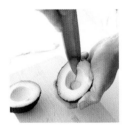

Cut in strips lengthwise and then cut in the opposite direction to dice.

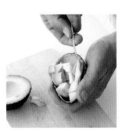

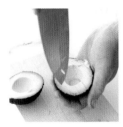

If you still believe that heated and processed food doesn't have a damaging effect on your body, try this test:

- Eat strictly raw food for a couple of weeks.
- Go back to eating your normal heated and processed food.
- How do you feel?

It's not pleasant! Believe me, I've tried it several times. When I first started eating raw, I immersed myself 100 percent. For a couple of weeks, I only ate raw food. Then, for mysterious reasons, I went back to my old way of living. It did not make me feel good! And I was forced to start all over again with raw food because my energy was gone, and it felt as if the normal food was practically sucking all the vitality and joy out of me.

I believed that my body was telling me what it needed, and I wasn't interested in fighting against inner conflicts and my own cravings. But why did my body tell me that it wanted nachos, cakes, and white bread? Slowly I realized that maybe it wasn't my body but my brain and old patterns that hankered for the "old" food, even though it definitely didn't benefit my quality of life or physical ability.

Now that I have turned 100 percent to raw food again and my body has had the chance to detoxify and find its balance, I can trust and recognize my body's signals. And believe me, it's not white sugar, burgers, ordinary chocolate, or heated, processed food that my body craves anymore.

It is fresh fruits, vegetables, nuts, and the like. I have never felt better, and food has never tasted so wonderful. But don't take my word for it—try this little test on your own.

Thanks!

Thanks to everyone who has inspired us, helped us, and supported us in this project. And thanks to my wonderful and beloved girlfriend Naja and to Vibeke's wonderful boys, Emilio and Oliver.

Index

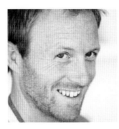

Jens Casupei helps people all over the world to be happy and live the life of their dreams. He ensures they achieve success in life by working with them physically, mentally, emotionally, and spiritually. He works with large and small groups as well as with individuals. Casupei designs and leads seminars on human development at the organization and management level for businesses. He has run management courses for some of the largest companies in Denmark. **www.casupei.com**

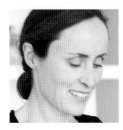

Vibeke Kaupert is a graphic designer from Denmark's Designschool, Institute of Visual Communication. "I'm crazy about raw food. The increased awareness, intuition, joy, health, and vitality that raw food has given me was something I wanted to share with the whole world." **www.kaupert.dk** and **www.vibekekaupert.com**